Practic
of t.

MW01141006

I.M.BALFOUR-LYNN

BSc, MRCP, FRCS(Ed), DHMSA
*Senior Registrar, Department of Child Health,
St Bartholomew's Hospital, London*

H.B.VALMAN

MD, FRCP, DCH, DRCOG
*Consultant Paediatrician to
Northwick Park Hospital
and Clinical Research Centre,
Harrow, Middlesex*

FIFTH EDITION

OXFORD

Blackwell Scientific Publications

LONDON EDINBURGH BOSTON

MELBOURNE PARIS BERLIN VIENNA

© 1971, 1973, 1975, 1979, 1993, by
Blackwell Scientific Publications
Editorial Offices:
Osney Mead, Oxford OX2 0EL
25 John Street, London, WC1N 2BL
23 Ainslie Place, Edinburgh EH3 6AJ
238 Main Street, Cambridge
  Massachusetts 02142, USA
54 University Street, Carlton
  Victoria 3053, Australia

Other Editorial Offices:
Librairie Arnette SA
2, rue Casimir-Delavigne
75006 Paris
France

Blackwell Wissenschafts-Verlag
Meinekestrasse 4
D-1000 Berlin 15
Germany

Blackwell MZV
Feldgasse 13
A-1238 Wien
Austria

First published 1971
as *Practical Neonatal Paediatrics*
Italian edition 1971
Second edition 1973
Third edition 1975
Fourth edition 1979
Reprinted 1986
Fifth edition 1993

Set by Semantic Graphics, Singapore
Printed and bound in Great Britain by
Hartnolls Ltd, Bodmin, Cornwall

DISTRIBUTORS

Marston Book Services Ltd
PO Box 87
Oxford OX2 0DT
(*Orders*: Tel: 0865 791155
      Fax: 0865 791927
      Telex: 837515)

USA
Blackwell Scientific Publications Inc.
238 Main Street
Cambridge, MA 02142
(*Orders*: Tel: 800 759–6102
      617 876–7000)

Canada
Times Mirror
Professional Publishing Ltd
130 Flaska Drive
Markham, Ontario L6G 1B8
(*Orders*: Tel: 800 268–4178
      416 470–6739)

Australia
Blackwell Scientific Publications
Pty Ltd
54 University Street,
Carlton, Victoria 3053
(*Orders*: Tel: 03 347–5552)

A catalogue record for this title
is available from the British Library

ISBN 0-632-03571-4

Library of Congress
Cataloging-in-Publication Data

Balfour-Lynn, I. M.
    Practical management of the
    newborn. — 5th ed./I.M. Balfour-Lynn,
    H.B. Valman.
        p.   cm.
    Rev. ed. of: Practical neonatal
    paediatrics/R.J.K. Brown, H.B. Valman.
    4th ed. 1979.
    Includes bibliographical references
    and index.
    ISBN 0-632-03571-4
    1. Infants (Newborn) — Diseases.
    2. Neonatology.   I. Valman, H.B.
    (Hyman Bernard)   II. Brown, R.J.K.
    (Roderick John Kilner). Practical
    neonatal paediatrics.   III. Title.
    [DNLM: 1. Infant Care.   2. Infant,
    Newborn.   3. Infant, Newborn,
    Diseases.   WS 420 B185p]
    RJ254.B76   1993
    618.92'01—dc20

Contents

Preface

It is over a decade since the fourth edition of *Practical Neonatal Paediatrics* was published. This book was intended to be a fifth edition but there have been so many changes that it warranted a new title. However the aims and character of the book have remained the same.

The book is primarily intended to teach medical and nursing staff how to look after newborn babies on the labour ward, postnatal ward and at home. The book assumes no previous paediatric experience and concentrates on practical issues rather than exhaustive details.

The first section deals with management of problems that may be anticipated before the baby is born.

The second section covers immediate emergencies at delivery as well as routine management of the baby, so should also be of use to midwives and junior obstetricians.

The final section deals with common problems that face the junior paediatricians and nurses on the postnatal wards. The emphasis is on early detection of illness and recognition of serious problems. It tells the reader what to do and when to call for help from senior colleagues. The book does not set out to cover detailed management of babies in the neonatal intensive care unit.

An increasing number of babies are discharged home after only 1–2 days to the care of the general practitioner and district midwife, and the book should also be a guide for them on the recognition and management of common neonatal problems.

NB: The masculine pronoun has been used throughout according to convention, but it also refers to the feminine gender.

Acknowledgements

We are grateful to Mr Andrew Fish for advice on obstetric matters included in the book. We are also grateful to Dr S.E. Holder for help with the sections on genetics. We would like to thank Dr Judith Stanton for reading the manuscript and making several helpful suggestions. We would particularly like to thank the nurses and midwives of the Neonatal Unit and Maternity Unit of Northwick Park Hospital for their advice. We would like to thank Mr Brian Mullan for his photographic work and baby Ryan and baby George for agreeing to have their photographs taken. We are grateful to the authors and publishers who have allowed us to reproduce material. Finally, we would like to thank our wives for their unstinting support and understanding during the preparation of this book.

List of Abbreviations

ACTH	adrenocorticotrophic hormone
ADH	antidiuretic hormone
AFP	α-fetoprotein
AIDS	acquired immune deficiency syndrome
ASD	atrial septal defect
BCG	bacille Calmette–Guérin
CAH	congenital adrenal hyperplasia
CBD	common bile duct
CCU	clean-catch urine
CDH	congenital dislocation of the hips
CF	cystic fibrosis
CMV	cytomegalovirus
CONI	Care Of Next Infant (scheme)
CSF	cerebrospinal fluid
CT	computerized tomography
CVB	chorionic villous biopsy
DD	homozygous D antigen
Dd	heterozygous D antigen
DJ	duodeno-jejunal (flexure)
DMSA	^{99m}Tc-Dimercaptosuccinate (scan)
DNA	deoxyribonucleic acid
DZ	dizygotic
EB	Epstein—Barr (virus)
ECG	electrocardiograph
ECM	external cardiac massage
EDTA	ethylenediaminetetra-acetic acid (edetic acid, edathamil)
EEG	electroencephalograph
EMLA	lignocaine 2.5%, prilocaine 2.5% cream
ETT	endotracheal tube
GBS	group B β-haemolytic *Streptococcus*
GOR	gastro-oesophageal reflux
G6PD	glucose-6-phosphate dehydrogenase
GTT	glucose tolerance test
Hb	haemoglobin

HBAg	hepatitis B antigen
HBsAg	hepatitis B surface antigen
HCt	haematocrit
HIV	human immunodeficiency virus
HMD	hyaline membrane disease
IC	intracardiac
IDM	infants of diabetic mothers
IgG	immunoglobulin G
IgM	immunoglobulin M
IM	intramuscular
IPPV	intermittent positive pressure ventilation
IQ	intelligence quotient
IRDS	idiopathic respiratory distress syndrome
IRT	immunoreactive trypsin
IT	intratracheal
ITP	idiopathic thrombocytopenic purpura
IV	intravenous
IUGR	intrauterine growth retardation
LBW	low birthweight
LP	lumbar puncture
LSD	lysergic acid diethylamide
MAP	mean arterial pressure
MCH	mean corpuscular haemoglobin
MCU	micturating cystourethrogram
MCV	mean corpuscular volume
MMR	measles/mumps/rubella
MRI	magnetic resonance imaging
MRSA	methicillin-resistant *Staphylococcus aureus*
MZ	monozygotic
NEC	necrotizing enterocolitis
NG	nasogastric
OA	oesophageal atresia
OFC	occipitofrontal circumference
PCV	packed cell volume
PDA	patent ductus arteriosus
PROM	prolonged rupture of membranes
RDS	respiratory distress syndrome
Rh	rhesus

SBR	serum bilirubin
SFD	small-for-dates
SID	sudden infant death (syndrome)
SLE	systemic lupus erythematosus
SPA	suprapubic aspirate
STD	sexually transmitted disease
SVT	supraventricular tachycardia
TAPVD	total anomalous pulmonary venous drainage
tds	three times a day
TGA	transposition of the great arteries
TOF	tracheo-oesophageal fistula
TPN	total parenteral nutrition
TSH	thyroid-stimulating hormone
TTN	transient tachypnoea of the newborn
UTI	urinary tract infection
UVC	umbilical venous catheter
VLBW	very low birthweight
VSD	ventricular septal defect
WCC	white cell count
ZIG	zoster immunoglobulin

Part 1
Anticipating Problems

1: Anticipating Problems —
Before Pregnancy

Many problems in the newborn arise unexpectedly, but it is sometimes possible to anticipate congenital malformations, illness and even death. Appropriate management may be made easier with some warning, even if the situation can not be prevented.

The first section of this book is concerned with anticipating and identifying situations that may adversely affect the baby. This first chapter deals with the period before conception.

PRE-EXISTING MATERNAL ILLNESS

Diabetes mellitus

Although the outlook has improved, diabetic mothers have a higher rate of complications and their babies have an increased mortality rate with deaths occurring late in the pregnancy. The incidence of congenital malformations is nearly doubled. The situation is made worse if the diabetes is poorly controlled, particularly if the mother has complications of the disease. The babies may be large (over 4.5 kg) and plethoric so there is a high rate of shoulder dystocia as they are often too large for the maternal pelvis. Respiratory distress similar to that found in premature babies is common. Because of islet-cell hyperplasia they are prone to hypoglycaemia which may be prolonged and management may be difficult for the first 48 hours (Chapter 14).

The diabetes is not always pre-existing. Sometimes glycosuria only develops during the pregnancy (gestational diabetes) and the diagnosis is confirmed by an abnormal glucose tolerance test (GTT). There are certain risk factors which indicate that the mother may develop gestational diabetes. These are known as 'potential diabetic' features and include obesity, a positive family history of diabetes, a history of unexplained intrauterine death, or previous infants with birthweights over 4.5 kg. If any of these factors are present, the mother should be screened with a GTT.

3

In addition, an apparently normal mother may have a baby with the features of an infant of a diabetic mother (noted above). The infant is managed as though the mother has diabetes and the mother is investigated in the next pregnancy for the presence of gestational diabetes.

Epilepsy
Pregnancy does not increase the risk of seizures, but poor compliance with treatment and overtiredness may cause problems. Seizures are more likely at the time of delivery due to hyperventilation and exhaustion. A seizure could theoretically cause fetal damage through hypoxia or through associated trauma.

Babies born to epileptic mothers tend to have lower birth-weights and smaller head circumferences, and the stillbirth rate is increased. Facial clefts and cleft palates are more common, but this is related to anticonvulsant therapy rather than the epilepsy itself. If the mother is taking anticonvulsant drugs through the pregnancy, the rate of congenital malformations is doubled (see p. 24).

Thyroid disease
The thyroid-stimulating autoantibodies which cause Grave's disease cross the placenta and can cause fetal hyperthyroidism manifest by persistent fetal tachycardia. The treatment is to give the mother anti-thyroid drugs which cross the placenta and prevent overactivity in the fetal thyroid. Thyrotoxicosis can also develop in the neonate within the first few days of life but sometimes it is not manifest for some weeks. The baby can have hyperactivity and tachycardia which may lead to heart failure. Other possible features are weight loss, irritability, goitre, exophthalmos, splenomegaly and petechiae.

Anti-thyroid drugs given to the mother can cause hypothyroidism in the fetus, although if the mother is rendered euthyroid the fetus is usually unaffected. The drugs can also cause a goitre if the fetus responds by producing more thyroid-stimulating hormone. Grave's disease tends to improve in the last trimester during which the mother is given a low maintenance dose.

Women with hypothyroidism have a higher rate of fetal loss. The babies must have their thyroid status checked as the mother may have had anti-thyroid antibodies present which can cross the placenta and cause fetal or transient neonatal hypothyroidism. The babies are otherwise normal.

Breastfed infants of mothers receiving anti-thyroid drugs should have thyroid function tests performed monthly.

Hypertension

Women with essential hypertension are more likely to develop pre-eclampsia (see p. 24), but hypertension without pre-eclampsia carries no extra risk to the fetus. None of the commonly used antihypertensive drugs are known to be teratogenic.

Thalassaemia

Thalassaemia is a haemoglobinopathy in which there is defective synthesis of the protein globin chains of the haemoglobin molecule. It is the commonest inherited blood disorder and particularly prevalent in Mediterranean races (especially Greeks, Cypriots, Italians) and Asians. The main types are alpha (α) and beta (β), depending on which globin chain is affected.

β-Thalassaemia

When the defect lies in the β-globin gene, it results in either β-thalassaemia major if the condition is homozygous or β-thalassaemia minor when heterozygous. The homozygous condition is very serious requiring life-long blood transfusions. The resultant iron overload damages the liver, pancreas, pituitary gland and heart and leads to a shortened life expectancy.

β-thalassaemia minor, on the other hand, is very common and results only in a microcytic hypochromic blood film with a very mild anaemia that requires no treatment. Diagnosis will often be made from the red cell indices performed with the full blood count taken from every woman during antenatal screening. Mean corpuscular volume (MCV) and mean corpuscular haemoglobin (MCH) are low but there is a relatively high red cell count. Confirmation is made by finding a raised HbA_2 level.

If both parents have β-thalassaemia trait then there is a one in four chance of the offspring having β-thalassaemia major. If the mother is known to have the trait before the pregnancy, then the father can be checked and prenatal diagnosis offered early in the pregnancy. However, if the mother is only diagnosed during routine antenatal screening, it will be late in the pregnancy before the status of the fetus is known.

α-Thalassaemia

There are normally four α-globin genes and the clinical picture depends on the number of genes that are deleted. If one or two genes are missing, the result is the mild condition α-thalassaemia trait. It is unlikely that the trait will have been detected before pregnancy unless the mother was screened for another reason, since the blood picture shows only a slightly low MCV and MCH but a normal haemoglobin level. However during pregnancy, the trait due to the two-gene deletion may cause a severe anaemia which would then be detected.

When three α-globin genes are missing the result is Haemoglobin H disease. Haemoglobin H disease (Hb H) is a chronic haemolytic anaemia, seen only in Greeks and Chinese. Finally, when all four genes are deleted, it causes α-thalassaemia major which is incompatible with life. The fetus develops *hydrops fetalis* and will only survive a few hours if born alive. This condition is quite common in South-East Asia.

If the mother is known to have an abnormality then the father's status must be checked. If the father is normal, and the mother has either α-thalassaemia trait or Hb H disease, then although the offspring may inherit the trait; they will not have any serious disease.

The real problem comes when both parents have the trait caused by a two-gene deletion. There is then a one in four risk of the child dying from *hydrops fetalis*, having inherited α-thalassaemia major. If the parents are at risk, then they must be referred for genetic counselling and prenatal diagnosis. It is preferable to diagnose the condition early in pregnancy in case intervention is necessary but this is only possible if the parents' condition is known before the pregnancy.

Sickle-cell disease

In this disorder of haemoglobin synthesis, the β-globin chain contains an incorrect amino acid. Under certain conditions such as low oxygen tension, acidosis or dehydration, the red blood cells are distorted into sickle shapes and can block small blood vessels. The disease results in a severe chronic haemolytic anaemia punctuated by acute crises of painful infarction, sequestration of blood in the spleen, and bone marrow failure. Clinical manifestations are seen after 6 months of life and affected children are at very great risk of infection due to poor splenic function. Inheritance is autosomal recessive, with homozygous HbSS resulting in sickle-cell anaemia and heterozygous HbAS producing the harmless sickle-cell trait. It is commonest in Afro-Caribbeans but is also seen in Indians, Saudi Arabians, Greeks and Cypriots.

If the mother has sickle-cell disease, there is a higher rate of fetal loss and preterm delivery as well as an increased risk to the mother herself. It is important to screen the father and if he is normal then the offspring will only have the trait.

Before pregnancy, the mother may not be aware of having sickle-cell trait and this may only be detected during antenatal screening. Again it is important to test the father as if he also has the trait then there is a one in four risk of the offspring having the full disease. The parents will then need genetic counselling and can be offered prenatal screening. If the father is normal, then the children will either have the trait or be normal themselves. In addition, high-risk populations can all be screened at birth by having cord blood estimations of HbS levels.

Idiopathic thrombocytopenic purpura (ITP)

In about half the cases, the maternal platelet antibodies cross the placenta causing thrombocytopenia in the neonate. The likelihood of the fetus being affected is related to the severity of the maternal disease, with 70% affected if the platelet count is less than 100×10^9/litre. The infant is at risk of an intracranial haemorrhage during a difficult delivery and there should be a low threshold for a Caesarean section. Intravenous immunoglobulin infusion causes a rise in platelet count in 80% of cases and in theory should cause a rise in the fetus as well but this is unproven. The platelet count in the newborn remains low for weeks but intervention is not usually necessary.

Systemic lupus erythematosus

There is an increased rate of fetal loss late in pregnancy due to hypertension and renal failure in the mother. Most babies born to mothers with systemic lupus erythematosus (SLE) are normal, but the fetus can be affected by maternal antibodies which cross the placenta. There may be haematological abnormalities such as haemolytic anaemia, leucopenia or thrombocytopenia but these are usually transient. There may also be cardiac abnormalities, usually a complete heart block which can be detected antenatally. Finally, neonatal lupus may only manifest itself by discrete discoid skin lesions on the face or scalp.

Myasthenia gravis

The maternal autoantibodies to acetylcholine neuromuscular receptors cross the placenta and in about 20% of cases cause transient neonatal myasthenia. This is manifest by hypotonia and weakness with poor sucking and a weak cry. Although usually wearing off after a few days, it may sometimes last for weeks. Occasionally the respiratory muscles are affected and then a small dose of anticholinesterase should be given.

SERIOUS SOCIAL PROBLEMS

There may be pre-existing social problems within the family which will put the newborn child at risk. Pregnancy and a new baby can certainly add to financial and emotional difficulties. The family may already be known to the social services department and sometimes case conferences will be held during the course of the pregnancy to ensure appropriate monitoring takes place once the child is born. Problems may only come to light during the pregnancy and attendance at antenatal clinic may be a good guide to the future care of the child. Unfortunately those who fail to attend are usually the mothers who need the most antenatal care. There are certain problems that should be highlighted.

Alcoholism

Babies born to alcoholic mothers may be born with fetal alcohol syndrome, the features of which are described on p. 117. Clinical manifestations may be noted if the mother is having four to six drinks/day but the full syndrome does not tend to appear until intake is at least eight to ten drinks/day. A 'drink' counts as one unit of alcohol which is a glass of wine, a single measure of spirits or half a pint of beer. There will also always be a serious concern that the mother will be unable to take care of the baby's needs.

Drug addiction

This is an increasing problem which is not always easy to recognize unless the mother is an intravenous drug abuser. If the mother uses dirty needles then there is a risk of septicaemia or transmission of HIV to the fetus (see p. 20). Babies of narcotic addicts are often small-for-dates, premature and more likely to have birth asphyxia. 60–90% of such babies suffer from withdrawal symptoms which can start anytime in the first week, but usually within 24–48 hours. They are jittery, irritable, sweaty, sneeze repeatedly and have a high-pitched scream. Many have diarrhoea and vomiting and they feed poorly. 10–20% have clonic fits. Treatment consists of sedation (usually with chlorpromazine) or small doses of opiates which are slowly withdrawn. Breastfeeding helps the baby through withdrawal as the milk will contain small amounts of narcotic. The child will be at risk of harm or neglect whilst the parents are under the influence of drugs once he or she is at home. Therefore close support will be needed from both the family and the community services.

The mother may have been abusing other drugs such as benzodiazepines, phenobarbitone or other sedatives. These tend to lead to a milder version of narcotic withdrawal in the baby. Cocaine abuse leads to a higher risk of congenital malformations, increased perinatal mortality and neurobehavioural impairment. Cannabis does not seem to cause harm to the fetus but is secreted into breast milk. LSD can cause chromosomal abnormalities and is associated with phocomelia (the hand or foot is attached directly to the trunk).

Smoking

Nicotine is also an addictive drug. There is a twofold increase in the rate of early spontaneous abortion in smokers. There is also a doubling in the rate of low birthweight infants. Part of this is accounted for by the association of smoking with premature labour. The influence of smoking on prematurity can not be separated from other adverse social factors that tend to be present in women who smoke through pregnancy. In babies of smokers who reach full term, the average weight is only 200 g less than babies of non-smokers. Recent evidence has shown that the baby's lung development is adversely affected *in utero* and this partially accounts for the increased incidence of asthma and respiratory infections amongst children of mothers who smoke.

Mental impairment

Problems with both the pregnancy and childcare can be anticipated when one or both parents have some form of mental impairment. This may be due to a serious psychiatric condition, for example a psychosis such as schizophrenia. In these cases, support will be needed from the psychiatrist, the community psychiatric nurse and social workers. The team will have to be sure the baby is safe with the mother and that the mother can cope with the child before allowing her to take the baby home. Once there, the baby must be closely monitored.

Similarly, when the mother has intellectual impairment with a very low IQ, extra support will be needed and much time put aside to teach basic parenting skills. Babies of such parents may suffer by neglect rather than by deliberate harm.

Schoolgirl mothers

Despite much publicity over contraception, in 1990 in England and Wales, there were over 1300 babies born to mothers aged under 16 years and over 4000 to 16-year-olds. These babies have an increased mortality rate and greater risk of prematurity, low birthweight, impaired growth and intellect. They are also at greater risk of child abuse. The mothers tend to book late and rarely attend antenatal clinics. Home circumstances are usually poor and great support is necessary.

Single mothers

In 1990 there were 200 000 babies born to single mothers in England and Wales (out of a total of just over 700 000). Almost half are unsupported which has obvious financial and social implications.

ILLNESS AND DEATH
IN A PREVIOUS CHILD

If a previous child has a serious illness or has died parents will be extremely anxious that the condition might recur. This is particularly true of a sudden infant death (SID) where there has been no obvious explanation as to why the baby died. When the new baby is born there may be an exacerbation of the parents' grieving and the mother may have difficulties with bonding and handling the baby. They will need continual reassurance that the baby is normal and close follow-up with an open-door policy to the paediatric department.

There is a programme currently running to help these parents look after and monitor their new baby. It is the CONI (care of next infant) scheme, which involves a multidisciplinary team including hospital paediatrician, health visitor, general practitioner and midwife. The baby is closely monitored with a daily symptom diary and daily or weekly weighing. In addition the child has an apnoea monitor and the parents are taught resuscitation techniques.

There is also the 'Baby Check' system developed in Cambridge and Melbourne in 1990. This is intended for use with all babies, not just those at high risk. There are 19 checks of important symptoms and signs that the parents can easily carry out. The score then indicates whether medical attention is needed and how urgently.

In some cases, a disease may have arisen spontaneously in the previous child. Specific screening may be possible once the baby is born or during early childhood. An example of this is a nephroblastoma, a tumour of the kidney that usually presents between the ages of 6 months and 3 years. It is probably present at birth and serial ultrasound examinations of the kidneys provide reassurance as well as early diagnosis.

Many conditions are inherited and genetic counselling can be offered to the parents. Advice can be given before the next pregnancy although the parents ought to have received counselling after the birth of the affected child.

GENETIC COUNSELLING BEFORE PREGNANCY

Multifactorial inheritance

In conditions with multifactorial inheritance, an empiric recurrence risk can be given although it will not be specific for a particular family. The parents can be told the risk but will then have to make their own decision as to whether or not to have another child. This is often an extremely difficult decision, largely dependent on the seriousness of the condition and whether treatment is possible. The issue over further children will only arise in relation to major congenital malformations and some examples are given below. Overall, the risks of recurrence are low but they increase if there is more than one affected child in the family (see Table 1.1).

Risks below one in 20 are considered low but this is obviously subjective. Should the parents decide to go ahead with another pregnancy, it may be possible to offer specific screening and early prenatal diagnosis (see p. 29).

Table 1.1 Risk of recurrence of congenital malformations in siblings (parents normal with one affected child).

Malformation	Risk to sibling
Neural tube defect	1 in 25*
Cleft lip and palate	1 in 25
Congenital heart disease	1 in 30
Renal agenesis	1 in 35
Clubfoot	1 in 50
Tracheo-oesophageal fistula	1 in 100

* There is geographical variation: risk is lower in South-East England and higher in Wales and Ireland.

Autosomal recessive conditions

In single-gene disorders more precise recurrence risks can be given depending on the type of inheritance. In autosomal recessive conditions such as cystic fibrosis or phenylketonuria, both parents must be carriers to have had an affected child. The risk is one in four for the next child having the disease and one in two that he or she will be a carrier of the defective gene. The chance of being completely normal is one in four. Autosomal recessive disorders tend to result in biochemical abnormalities often involving only a single enzyme. The carrier may be asymptomatic, as in cystic fibrosis, and the carrier status will only be revealed after the birth of an affected child. Sometimes carriers have a mild form of the disease such as sickle-cell trait or β-thalassaemia minor and they may be aware of this before the first pregnancy.

Autosomal dominant conditions

In autosomal dominant conditions, one of the parents is affected phenotypically even though he or she only carries a single copy of the defective gene (heterozygous). Examples are achondroplasia, Marfan's syndrome and neurofibromatosis. Assuming the other parent is normal, the risk to children will be one in two. The disorders tend to result in structural abnormalities that are obvious; however the clinical severity may vary between individual members of the same family.

The parents will usually seek advice before having their first child. Some autosomal dominant conditions arise in offspring of normal parents and these are due to a spontaneous mutation in the sperm or egg. In these cases, the risk of recurrence is very low.

Sex-linked conditions

The other type of inherited disorders are the sex-linked conditions. The mother carries an abnormal gene on one of her X chromosomes. Assuming the father is normal, then there is a one in two chance of a boy having the condition, and a one in two chance of a girl being a carrier. Girls will either be normal or be carriers, whereas boys will either have the full condition or be

normal. Examples are Duchenne muscular dystrophy and haemophilia. An affected father and normal mother will produce
either normal sons or daughters who are carriers.

Chromosomal disorders

With chromosomal disorders, it may also be possible to provide
recurrence risks. The exact chromosome abnormality of the child
and parents needs to be known, particularly in the case of
Down's syndrome (Chapter 9). If the child has Trisomy 21 then
the risk of having another child with a chromosomal abnormality
is 1% for a mother under 37 years of age. Older mothers have a
higher risk of having a child with Down's syndrome, and if in
addition they already have one affected child, then the risk of
them having another is double that expected for their age.

If the child with Down's syndrome has a translocation that
arose spontaneously then there is no extra risk for other children.
If however the translocation was passed on by one of the parents
who is a carrier, the risk is 2% if the father carries 14/21
translocation, 10% if the mother carries 14/21 translocation and
100% if either parent carries 21/21 translocation. Finally, if the
child has mosaic Down's, in which some of the cells are normal
whilst some cells have an extra chromosome 21, then there is no
extra risk that future children will have Down's syndrome.

Carrier status

It may be important to test prospective parents for carrier status.
This may be relatively simple, with the potential for screening
whole populations, for example with sickle-cell disease or thalassaemia. However, testing for carriers is usually only done in
families who are known to be at risk of a particular disease. In
some instances, the parents are known to be carriers (if, for
example, they have had a child with an autosomal recessive
condition). Often, however, a couple are considering starting a
family when one of them has a positive family history. For
example, the brother of someone with cystic fibrosis will want to
know whether he is a carrier. If he is, he will then want to know
whether his wife is a carrier, as this would give them a one in
four chance of having an affected child.

With new techniques of DNA analysis using gene probes, it is now possible to detect the majority of carriers of cystic fibrosis in the population. Examples of autosomal recessive diseases that are amenable to DNA analysis are cystic fibrosis, congenital adrenal hyperplasia, galactosaemia and phenylketonuria. It is also important in sex-linked disorders, as many female relatives in a family may be carriers and able to pass on the disease. Some of these carriers can also now be detected, for example in Duchenne muscular dystrophy, haemophilia, fragile X syndrome and retinitis pigmentosa.

Parental age

Although Down's syndrome is the commonest example, maternal age affects the incidence of several major chromosomal abnormalities. Older mothers have a greater incidence of children with other autosomal trisomies, for example Trisomy 18 (Edwards' syndrome) and Trisomy 13 (Patau syndrome), as well as sex-chromosome disorders such as 47,XXY (Klinefelter syndrome) and 47,XXX. Paternal age has little effect on the risk of chromosomal abnormalities, but older fathers have an increased risk of producing new autosomal dominant mutations leading to disorders such as achondroplasia and Marfan's syndrome.

Parental consanguinity

Over 50% of the Pakistani community in the UK marry their first cousins, and there are often marriages between second cousins and between uncles and nieces. Consanguineous marriages also take place to a lesser extent amongst Bangladeshis. Indians, who are predominantly Hindu, do not marry within the family.

Because of a shared genetic background, there is an increased chance that the parents will be carriers of the same recessive genes which results in an increased incidence of autosomal recessive diseases. There is also an increase in multifactorial abnormalities and in severe mental retardation. The risk of a major congenital abnormality is doubled, and with a positive family history it is higher still. There is no effect on dominantly-inherited or X-linked disorders.

It is insensitive to blame consanguineous parents when they

have a baby with an inherited condition. However, both the parents and the extended family should be offered genetic counselling when the presence of a lethal or serious recessive gene within the family is revealed by the birth of an affected child.

FURTHER READING

Black J (1990) *Child Health in a Multicultural Society.* British Medical Association, London.

De Swiet M (1989) *Medical Disorders in Obstetric Practice.* Blackwell Scientific Publications, Oxford.

Kingston H (1989) *ABC of Clinical Genetics.* British Medical Association, London.

Morley CJ, Thornton AJ, Cole TJ, Hewson PH & Fowler MA (1991) Baby Check: a scoring system to grade the severity of acute systemic illness in babies under 6 months old. *Archives of Disease in Childhood,* **66**: 100–5.

2: Anticipating Problems — During Pregnancy

We are now concerned with risk factors arising or identified during the pregnancy which may adversely affect the baby. The problem may be apparent either in the mother or the fetus.

MATERNAL

Acute infections
Any severe infection can cause fetal death or premature birth, and if the mother is unwell for some time then fetal growth may be affected due to disturbance in nutrition. In some infections, the mother may not be too unwell but the infecting agent may cause serious harm to the fetus.

Bacteria
It is unusual for bacteria to cross the placenta and infect the fetus. The commonest bacterial infections of pregnancy are due

to Gram-negative organisms, particularly *Escherichia coli*, which cause an acute lower urinary tract infection or acute pyelonephritis. With appropriate antibiotic treatment the fetus is not affected but there is an associated increased incidence of urinary infection in the newborn.

Recent research has suggested that chronic carriage of certain microorganisms in the mother's genital tract may be associated with recurrent preterm labour or stillbirths. This particularly applies to *Chlamydia*, and to a lesser extent *Mycoplasma*. The implication is that microbiological screening may be useful in women considered to be high risk.

There are certain bacterial infections that may cause serious problems to the fetus if acquired during the pregnancy.

Congenital listeriosis is caused by the Gram-positive *Listeria monocytogenes*. In almost half the cases the mother simply has a flu-like illness with a mild fever and the diagnosis is often made retrospectively after the birth of an affected child. In other cases the mother has a recurrent febrile illness with malaise, headache, backache, abdominal pain and sometimes sore throat, conjunctivitis and diarrhoea. In early pregnancy it can cause abortion, whilst in later pregnancy it causes stillbirths and premature labour within a week of infection. It has recently been associated with eating soft unpasteurized cheeses such as Brie and Camembert during pregnancy. The clue to diagnosis in the baby is thick dark amniotic fluid that is often incorrectly thought to be meconium. Remember, premature babies do not pass meconium *in utero*. Early features are respiratory distress due to pneumonia, diarrhoea with mucus, convulsions, and discrete rose or pustular spots on the skin and back of the throat. A late form exists, in which the baby of a healthy mother develops meningitis after the fifth day but this is not a congenital infection. Diagnosis is confirmed by culturing amniotic fluid, superficial skin swabs, ear fluid or blood. Treatment consists of high-dose intravenous ampicillin and the high mortality is usually due to delayed diagnosis.

Pulmonary tuberculosis had become an uncommon complication of pregnancy but there has been an upsurge in the disease, particularly in the immigrant communities in the UK. With the use of antituberculous drugs, the disease no longer has a deleterious effect on the pregnancy for either mother or fetus. Certain of the drugs, however, should be avoided in early pregnancy because of potential teratogenic effects, these include streptomycin, rifampicin and pyrazinamide. Although tuberculosis rarely affects the fetus by transplacental passage, the baby has a 50% risk of contracting the disease after delivery unless suitable prophylaxis is given. If the organism is sensitive to isoniazid, the newborn should be given isoniazid for at least 3 months to prevent infection. In addition the baby should receive isoniazid-resistant BCG immediately to allow immunity to develop. Should the infant develop the disease, it does not manifest itself for about 6 weeks. There is failure to thrive with poor feeding, weight loss, vomiting and hepatosplenomegaly. Without treatment, the child will die from widespread miliary tuberculosis.

Since antituberculosis antibodies are IgM, the infant cannot acquire immunity from the mother as the IgM is too large to cross the placenta. If the mother has had tuberculosis in the past the child should be given BCG immunization shortly after birth. Some health authorities offer routine BCG to all babies from high-risk groups once they have left the maternity hospital. If the BCG immunization is delayed, it should not be given until a tuberculin skin test (e.g. Mantoux test) is shown to be negative.

Gonococcal conjunctivitis is caused by gonococcal infection transmitted from the mother's genital tract at birth. It causes an acute purulent conjunctivitis apparent within 5 days. It can also involve the cornea and cause blindness. Systemic manifestations of gonococcus, including pneumonia, meningitis and arthritis are also described. Treatment is chloramphenicol eye ointment applied half-hourly at first and then every 2 hours for 3 days. Intravenous benzylpenicillin should also be given for 7 days but cultures must confirm antibiotic sensitivity as the gonococcus may be penicillin-resistant. If the mother has a vaginal discharge at the time of delivery and microscopy shows the presence of Gram-negative diplococci, treatment should be started without delay on the assumption that gonococcus will be isolated (see also p. 197).

Congenital syphilis is now rare in the UK due to screening of all mothers in the antenatal clinic combined with early treatment. In half the cases the child contracts the disease, and in another third of cases the fetus is stillborn. If severely affected, the child may have clinical features present at birth. These include hepato-splenomegaly with jaundice, bloody and purulent nasal discharge, maculopapular skin rash and anaemia. An X-ray of the long bones shows a thickened dense epiphyseal line with an adjacent area of rarefaction. However, the child may appear normal at birth but over a month or so may fail to thrive and may develop some of the above features. In another group, the child manifests no symptoms for years until he develops late sequelae from chronic infection. The manifestations include deformities of the bones and teeth, corneal inflammation, nerve deafness and neurosyphilis leading to psychomotor retardation. Diagnosis is confirmed by detecting specific IgM. Treatment is 2 weeks of high-dose benzylpenicillin.

Viruses
Although many maternally acquired viruses cross the placenta, most of them cause little harm to the fetus. Some however can have serious consequences and the most important viruses implicated are rubella, cytomegalovirus (CMV), varicella zoster, HIV and human parvovirus B19. Viruses may also be acquired by the newborn baby from the mother at the time of delivery, for example herpes simplex, varicella zoster, HIV, enteroviruses and hepatitis B.

Rubella almost invariably damages the fetus if acquired in the first trimester. Defects are less likely after 13 weeks and rare after 17 weeks gestation. Its teratogenic effects are outlined on p. 114. It is also associated with an increased rate of abortion and still-births.

Cytomegalovirus is the other virus that has teratogenic effects (see p. 114). Transplacental infection occurs in 30–40% cases and only 10% of infected fetuses are severely damaged. Again there is an association with abortions and stillbirths.

Varicella zoster can also harm the fetus but congenital varicella syndrome is fortunately rare. The main effects are mental deficiency with seizures, chorioretinitis, poor fetal growth, limb hypoplasia and severe cutaneous scarring.

Varicella acquired in the baby at the time of delivery can cause a severe chickenpox infection which has an appreciable mortality. The baby is most at risk if the mother has chickenpox spots that appear less than 5 days before delivery or less than 7 days after the birth. The baby should receive anti-varicella zoster immunoglobulin (ZIG) 0.5 ml intramuscularly. If he still develops chickenpox then acyclovir may be appropriate. If the mother develops zoster infection (shingles) then the baby is protected as the mother will have had chickenpox in the past and the fetus will have acquired transplacental antibodies (see also p. 201).

Human immunodeficiency virus (HIV). Vertical transmission of HIV infection is now recognized and the number of babies affected is likely to increase progressively. About 30–40% of children born to HIV-positive mothers are infected with the virus, either before, during or shortly after birth. There is no evidence that HIV causes congenital malformations. HIV infection is difficult to diagnose as the maternal antibodies may persist for up to 18 months. 25% of HIV-positive children develop AIDS by the age of 1 year and 80% by 4 years. A small proportion present with sudden onset of a rapidly fulminating disease. However, many children remain symptom-free for years and present with non-specific illnesses such as recurrent infection, diarrhoea, lymphadenopathy and failure to thrive.

Human parvovirus B19 is either subclinical or causes a mild rubella-like illness in pregnancy. Transplacental infection occurs in a third of the cases but most of these babies are unaffected. However 10% of the infected babies develop severe hydrops fetalis and are stillborn or abort, particularly if infection occurs in the second trimester. A marker of poor fetal outcome is a raised maternal serum α-fetoprotein as it is associated with an aplastic crisis in the fetus.

Herpes simplex is important because genital herpes can be transmitted to the baby during delivery. Caesarean section is recommended if the lesions are active at the time but if quiescent, or if
there is only a past history of herpes then vaginal delivery is safe.
If the baby acquires herpes, it may only be localized to the eyes,
skin or mucous membranes. However, it can cause a severe
systemic infection with hepatosplenomegaly and jaundice,
meningoencephalitis and potentially fatal disseminated intra-
vascular coagulation. Intravenous acyclovir is the treatment.

Hepatitis A does not appear to have any adverse effect on the
fetus, although there are some reports that it is associated with
preterm delivery. There is a small risk that the baby could
become infected from faecal contamination during delivery. If the
mother still has hepatitis A at birth, it is prudent to give the baby
2 ml of standard immunoglobulin intramuscularly.

Hepatitis B can lead to preterm delivery if the mother has the
acute infection in the third trimester. The major problem is that
the mother may infect the baby, either vertically (i.e. *in utero* or
during delivery) or horizontally (in early childhood). There is a
tendency for the newborn of infected mothers to become chronic
carriers, and up to 40% of the world's chronic carriers acquire
the disease this way. A carrier is defined as a patient who is
HBsAg-positive for over 6 months.
    There are several maternal risk factors for vertical transmission:
1 Acute infection in the third trimester or up to 5 weeks post-
partum.
2 A chronic carrier with a high-titre HBsAg who is HBeAg-
positive. There is a 90% risk that the baby will develop evidence
of infection as presence of the 'e' antigen indicates active viral
replication.
3 A chronic carrier who is seronegative for both HBeAG and
anti-HBe (the antibodies against the 'e' antigen). The babies are
at particularly high risk of acute, even fulminant, hepatitis B.
4 Mother originates from the Far East.
    The majority of babies who acquire the infection are asympto-
matic but become HBsAg-positive between 6 weeks and 4 months.

A small proportion have a mild clinical illness after the second week with jaundice and hepatomegaly. Finally, a very small percentage develop a fulminant hepatitis and die of massive liver necrosis.

Development of chronic carrier status is uncommon in babies whose mothers have acute hepatitis B in the third trimester. It is also uncommon in babies of those mothers who are chronic carriers but have evidence of low viral replication (i.e. are HBeAg-negative or anti-HBe-positive).

On the other hand, the majority of babies of HBeAg-positive mothers become chronic carriers. There is also a correlation of development of carrier status with a high titre of HBsAg in the cord blood. The concern over carrier status is due to the fact that 50% of longstanding chronic carriers will die of hepatitis B-related liver disease.

All mothers attending antenatal clinics who are at high risk should be screened for hepatitis B. Many urban hospitals now screen all mothers as it is not always easy to identify those at risk. Risk factors include those who originate from endemic areas even if they are born in the UK (e.g. Far East, South-East Asia, Middle East and Asia), women with occupational exposure, or those who have had multiple blood transfusions, tattoos or a history of intravenous drug abuse.

There are no firm recommendations for prophylaxis, but here are some guidelines:

1 If the mother has current active hepatitis B or is a HBeAg-positive carrier the baby should receive both passive and active immunization. Immediately after birth, the baby must be given 0.5 ml of intramuscular specific hepatitis B immunoglobulin. He should also receive one of the hepatitis B vaccines within 48 hours of birth and boosters 1 month and 6 months after the first dose.

2 If the mother is a HBeAg-positive carrier but is also anti-HBe-positive, then only the vaccine is necessary.

3 If the mother is a HBeAg-negative carrier and has become anti-HBe-positive, it has recently been recommended that the baby should receive the vaccine, whereas it was previously suggested that no prophylaxis was necessary.

Both mother and baby should be isolated and there is no

contraindication to breastfeeding. The children should be followed up in out-patients to check their antibody status.

Other viruses. Many other viruses have been implicated in causing congenital malformations and fetal death. These include mumps, influenza, EB virus, coxsackie A4, B3 and B4 (the latter two are thought to cause fetal myocarditis), measles and poliomyelitis. These effects however are rarely seen and the evidence is often circumstantial.

Chlamydia

Chlamydia trachomatis is often asymptomatic but may be manifest in the mother by vaginal discharge or a history of non-specific urethritis. If she has a genital infection, perinatal transmission occurs in 25–50% cases and may result in neonatal conjunctivitis or pneumonia. Intrauterine infection is unusual unless there is prolonged rupture of membranes. The baby should be treated with both oral erythromycin and tetracycline eye ointment for 14 days if conjunctivitis is present (see p. 197).

Parasites

Both toxoplasmosis and malaria are important in pregnancy.

Congenital toxoplasmosis follows a primary infection in the mother. Transplacental infection is less common in the first trimester but should it occur the results are more severe than when the fetus is infected later in the pregnancy. Over 70% of infected newborn show no overt clinical signs and although some of these babies remain asymptomatic, some will develop late damage to the central nervous system (see p. 114), therefore all infected children require long-term follow-up.

Malaria may infect the placenta and cause abortion, stillbirth and growth retardation. The parasites can also cross the placenta, particularly if it is the mother's first infection. The neonate requires prolonged treatment, usually with chloroquine. Mothers should be encouraged to take prophylaxis if travelling to endemic areas as malaria has a predilection for pregnancy.

Pre-eclampsia
This is a disease of the last trimester and is more common in mothers under 20 or over 35 years of age or in the case of twin pregnancies. In longstanding cases with proteinuria, the fetus may be growth-retarded and there is a risk of intrauterine death. Sometimes premature delivery is necessary for the sake of both the mother and baby. Although the babies are often small, they tend to cope better than other babies of an equivalent size.

Prescribed drugs in pregnancy
Adverse effects on the fetus have been described in association with over 40 drugs. This suggests that no drug should be given in pregnancy unless there is a strong clinical indication. At the beginning of pregnancy, and preferably before conception, all the drugs prescribed should be reviewed to avoid unnecessary risk. The actual outcome may vary according to gestational age of the fetus who is most at risk during the first trimester — the period of organogenesis. Some drugs are essential to treat maternal disease but it may be possible to reduce the dose or substitute a safer alternative.

Some drugs have proven teratogenic effects and are definitely contraindicated. Thalidomide caused severe limb defects in over 10 000 children when it was used in the 1960s. Diethylstilboestrol caused female babies to develop carcinoma of the vagina or cervix after puberty. Cytotoxic chemotherapy causes gross congenital malformations. Methotrexate which may be used for psoriasis causes skull and rib defects as well as missing digits. Radioisotopes and all forms of ionizing radiation in early pregnancy cause multiple anomalies, and are associated with development of leukaemia in later childhood. Progestogens (which were used for threatened abortion) cause virilization of females. Live viral vaccines such as rubella, measles and poliomyelitis are also completely contraindicated.

Many other drugs cause a variety of effects but may still need to be used. High doses of barbiturates and phenytoin in epileptic mothers are associated with an increased incidence of cleft lip and palate, congenital heart disease, fingernail hypoplasia and poor growth, although the exact contribution of the drugs is uncertain. Sodium valproate can cause neural tube defects, cardiac anomalies and facial defects.

Tetracycline may affect bone growth and induce staining and possibly hypoplasia of the tooth enamel. Aminoglycosides (e.g. streptomycin, neomycin) may cause congenital nerve deafness. Long-acting sulphonamides given shortly before delivery may cause severe jaundice by competing with bilirubin for binding sites on serum albumin. Chloroquine may cause retinal damage. Quinine can cause hydrocephalus, heart defects and limb abnormalities. Isoniazid can cause convulsions due to pyridoxine deficiency. The penicillins are safe.

Prednisolone given throughout pregnancy may cause growth retardation, but dexamethasone may help lung maturation in premature labour.

Methyldopa and hydralazine are safe drugs for control of maternal hypertension. However ganglion-blockers cause meconium ileus; β-blockers (e.g. propanalol, labetalol) can cause respiratory depression, bradycardia and hypoglycaemia; captopril causes high fetal mortality in animal studies; sodium nitroprusside is also toxic to the fetus. Whilst frusemide is safe, chlorothiazide diuretics may cause thrombocytopenic purpura.

Oral hypoglycaemic drugs can cause neonatal hypoglycaemia, thrombocytopenia, and may be associated with congenital anomalies. Insulin is the safest treatment for maternal diabetes.

Long-term treatment of maternal venous thrombosis is controversial. Warfarin given in the first trimester is associated with a low but definite incidence of teratogenesis, causing cartilage and bone anomalies. In later pregnancy it has also been suggested that it may cause repeated small intracerebral haemorrhages that lead to optic atrophy, microcephaly and mental retardation. Some obstetricians no longer use warfarin at all. Heparin does not cross the placenta but has been associated with increased fetal morbidity after long-term use.

Anti-thyroid drugs can cause neonatal hypothyroidism or a goitre. High-dose salicylates can lead to neonatal jaundice in a similar way to sulphonamides. Salicylates and indomethacin can also lead to premature closure of the ductus arteriosus as they inhibit prostaglandin synthetase. Lithium can cause cardiac malformations. Vitamin D can cause hypercalcaemia, and in very large doses has been associated with supravalvular aortic stenosis, an elfin facies and mental retardation.

The use of ritodrine to prevent premature labour can lead to fetal tachycardia and hyperglycaemia. Prolonged use of oxytocin to promote labour is associated with hyponatraemia in the neonate due to fluid overload. This is caused by the drug's antidiuretic hormone-like effect as well as accompanying overuse of hypo-osmolar 5% glucose during labour. Pethidine given shortly before delivery can lead to respiratory depression in the baby. Anaesthetic agents given for a Caesarean section will also cause transient respiratory depression.

Rhesus incompatibility

Red blood cells contain various antigens, including those of the rhesus (Rh) system. Most relevant is the D antigen which is determined by the rhesus genes on one pair of chromosomes. If the individual has the D antigen he is blood group rhesus-positive, and he may be homozygous (DD) or heterozygous (Dd). If the baby has no D antigen, he is rhesus-negative with dd genotype. 85% of the population in the UK are rhesus-positive. Rhesus incompatibility can arise only when the mother is rhesus-negative and the father rhesus-positive, in which case if the father is homozygous all children will be rhesus-positive, whereas if he is heterozygous then there is only a 50% chance of the child being rhesus-positive.

During a normal pregnancy, very few fetal blood cells pass into the maternal circulation. However, during labour, as the placenta begins to tear away from its attachment to the uterine wall, a significant number of fetal blood cells may pass across to the mother. If the mother is rhesus-negative, and the fetus rhesus-positive, the rhesus-positive fetal red cells may stimulate production of maternal anti-D antibodies. There will be no effect on this fetus, but problems may arise in a subsequent pregnancy. The maternal anti-D antibodies are predominantly of the IgG class so they can cross the placenta and enter the fetal circulation. If this fetus is also rhesus-positive, the antibodies will cause agglutination and haemolysis of the fetal red cells which can have serious consequences, namely haemolytic disease of the newborn.

The infant may be affected in three ways although these are not always totally distinct. In the most severe form the infant is stillborn or grossly oedematous with ascites and heart failure (hydrops fetalis). The second manifestation is severe or moderate jaundice that develops soon after birth, and may be accompanied by a degree of haemolytic anaemia. Finally, the infant may simply be affected with mild jaundice but develop anaemia in the first few weeks.

All women have their blood group screened at the first visit to the antenatal clinic. All rhesus-negative women should have anti-D antibody titres checked, and if no antibodies are present this is repeated at 28, 32 and 36 weeks. If it is the first pregnancy there should not be a problem although the mother may have been sensitized after a previous miscarriage without even being aware of this. If antibodies are present at the first check, then levels need to be repeated more often. High titres or a sudden rise indicate the fetus is at risk, but this alone is not a reliable guide to the state of the fetus.

Aminocentesis at around 32 and 34 weeks will be necessary in some cases, and the level of bilirubin staining as well as antibody levels in the amniotic fluid can be calculated. This may predict the presence of a severely affected fetus and a need for early delivery. It will also avoid unnecessary delivery of a premature infant who may not be too badly affected. Fetal haemoglobin can also be estimated from samples taken by cordocentesis (see p. 32).

In a critical situation, when the baby is still very premature (usually less than 30 weeks gestation), instead of delivering the baby it may be safer to perform an intrauterine transfusion. This is done via the umbilical cord under ultrasound control.

The whole situation can usually be avoided by preventing sensitization of the mother after delivery of her first rhesus-positive child. Within 48 hours of delivery, she should be give an intramuscular injection of anti-D immunoglobulin (500 units). This will destroy the fetal red cells with their D antigen before the mother produces her own anti-D antibodies. It will not work if she has already produced antibodies earlier in the pregnancy but this is unusual. The size of the fetomaternal transfusion can be estimated using the Kleihauer test and if this shows a high fetal red cell count in the mother's blood, a larger dose of anti-D immunoglobulin is given. If the mother and baby are also ABO incompatible (mother is group O and baby group A or B), future rhesus incompatibility will not be a problem. This is because the fetal red cells are destoyed in the maternal circulation by the mother's anti-A or anti-B antibodies before they can stimulate production of anti-D.

Whenever a rhesus-negative mother has a baby, cord blood should be sent for determination of the baby's blood group, haemoglobin, bilirubin and a Coombs' test. The Coombs' test indicates the presence of red cells coated with antibody, so a positive result proves the baby has been affected. A severely affected infant (Coombs' positive and cord Hb < 12 g/dl or cord bilirubin > 70 µmol/l) will need an immediate exchange transfusion to raise the Hb and remove red cells damaged by antibody. Premature babies are at greater risk from high bilirubin levels so exchange transfusions are carried out more readily. In less severe cases, the serum bilirubin should be checked every 8 hours and phototherapy started early. For further details on treatment of jaundice see p. 173. In cases that do not receive an exchange transfusion, the Hb may continue to fall for several weeks and it should be checked weekly for the first 6 weeks. If the Hb falls below 7 g/dl a top-up transfusion with fresh blood may be necessary.

Due to successful prevention, rhesus incompatibility is not seen very often now and it may be more appropriate for mothers to be managed in specialist centres, particularly if she has had a previous severely affected child or stillbirth.

Hydramnios
Hydramnios or polyhydramnios is a condition in which there is excessive liquor. It occurs in one in 200 pregnancies and tends to arise after the 30th week but the cause is often obscure. It is recognized by a larger than expected abdomen and there are increased fetal movements. The membranes are more prone to rupture, hence premature labour is common. Malpresentations and cord prolapse also occur often. Maternal causes include

diabetes mellitus as well as cardiovascular and renal problems. Maternal hypertension may arise secondary to the hydramnios. There are also several fetal anomalies that lead to hydramnios, hence its importance as a warning sign.

Anencephaly (see p. 102) is one cause and it is thought the hydramnios is due to a lack of ADH (antidiuretic hormone) in the baby that leads to excess fluid production, as well as a lack of fetal swallowing. Oesophageal atresia also leads to hydramnios due to lack of fetal swallowing (see p. 102). Other causes include high intestinal obstructions of the pylorus, duodenum and jejunum as well as meconium ileus (Chapter 13), congenital diaphragmatic hernia (Chapter 5), spina bifida (see p. 101) and hydrops fetalis. A normal twin pregnancy is another cause. Careful ultrasound scanning is needed whenever hydramnios occurs.

Oligohydramnios
Oligohydramnios is a lack of amniotic fluid. It is uncommon and when it occurs the cause is usually unknown. It may arise after prolonged or repetitive episodes of uteroplacental insufficiency that give rise to intrauterine growth retardation. It may also accompany anomalies of the fetal urinary tract, in particular the renal agenesis of Potter's syndrome (see p. 109). As a secondary consequence of being compressed, the fetus may develop talipes, ankylosis of several joints, torticollis and even scoliosis. In addition, amniotic adhesions may attach to the fetus and lead to skin defects over bony prominences such as the malleoli, trochanters and shoulders. Scalp defects may also occur. The adhesions can even cause strangulation of limbs leading to amputation. Strangulation of the umbilical cord resulting in intrauterine death has also been described. Oligohydramnios may also be due to premature rupture of membranes and in these cases the baby may develop pulmonary hypoplasia which is usually fatal (see p. 55). There is also a risk of ascending infection.

FETAL

Prenatal diagnosis
There are an ever-increasing number of fetal abnormalities that can be detected early in pregnancy. There are now a number of

techniques available to the obstetrician although some are only possible in specialist referral centres. Fetal problems may be detected during routine antenatal screening performed in all pregnancies. These involve non-invasive tests such as ultrasound scanning and maternal blood screening. A disorder may also be found after specific testing initiated following previous problems or when an abnormality is picked up on routine screening. These tests are more invasive and may involve sampling of fetal tissue. They include chorionic villous biopsy, amniocentesis and fetal blood sampling.

Non-invasive screening
Ultrasound examination is routinely performed on all mothers at around 18 weeks gestation and is now the mainstay of antenatal screening for major congenital abnormalities. Over 200 different fetal anomalies have now been diagnosed *in utero* and in some centres up to 85% of anomalies can be detected prenatally by this method. An early scan will pick up major anomalies and give the gestational age of the fetus. It will also diagnose twin pregnancies and should be done at 16–18 weeks. There would appear to be no risk to the mother or fetus.

If there is any problem, then a detailed anomaly scan should be performed and this is best done at 20 weeks. It will measure various parameters of fetal size and visualize the head (including brain and ventricles), lips, spine, heart and chest, diaphragm, abdominal wall and cord insertion, intra-abdominal masses, kidneys and bladder, genitalia, limbs and digits. It can also determine placental size and position and the number of vessels in the umbilical cord.

Examples of abnormalities that can be diagnosed are neural tube defects, hydrocephaly and microcephaly, cleft lip and palate, cardiac defects, hydrops fetalis, congenital diaphragmatic herniae, renal disease such as agenesis or hydronephrosis, abdominal wall defects (exomphalos, gastroschisis), and various skeletal and limb anomalies.

If an abnormality is found, serial scans may be necessary to monitor progress. In addition, referral for specialist scanning may be required, particularly for cardiac defects. Counselling is necessary for the parents who may opt for a termination of pregnancy depending on the nature of the condition and their personal beliefs. Many defects are amenable to surgery and in these cases, planned delivery of the baby at a neonatal surgical centre is preferable.

Maternal serum a-fetoprotein (AFP) levels can be determined, and in some districts this is offered as a routine screen for neural tube defects. AFP is produced by the fetus and crosses the placenta into the maternal circulation. It is also detectable in amniotic fluid which it reaches by diffusing through fetal skin in the first trimester. Later on, it is excreted in the fetal urine into amniotic fluid. At 16–18 weeks gestation, raised maternal AFP indicates there may be an anencephaly or open spina bifida. There is an overlap with normal values so false positives occur. If abnormal, the AFP should be repeated and a detailed ultrasound scan performed. Certain other fetal anomalies may also give rise to a raised AFP and these include anterior abdominal wall defects and teratomas.

Low maternal AFP levels are associated with Down's syndrome as well as other chromosomal abnormalities. The risk of Down's syndrome can be calculated from the AFP level and maternal age. This is more accurate if maternal serum levels of unconjugated oestriol (reduced in Down's) and human chorionic gonadotrophin (raised in Down's) are taken into account. This combination of tests is often called the Bart's test (after St Bartholomew's Hospital, London) or the Triple test. Diagnosis will need to be confirmed by amniocentesis but risk calculation will enable a greater detection of cases of Down's syndrome with a lower rate of amniocentesis. The main use is for screening younger mothers who are not normally considered at high risk, even though 60% of babies with Down's syndrome are born to mothers under 37 years of age. The Bart's test is not yet widely available.

Invasive testing
Chorionic villous biopsy (CVB) provides fetal trophoblast cells. Sampling has traditionally been done through the cervix but a

transabdominal route under ultrasound guidance is now coming into favour. There is a 3–4% risk of fetal loss as well as a risk of intrauterine infection and limb abnormalities. Its main advantage is that it can be performed at 9–11 weeks so that late termination of pregnancy is avoided. Information can be provided on the fetal karyotype, including the sex of the fetus, within 48 hours. Detection of minor chromosomal anomalies takes 3–4 weeks. CVB is particularly useful when there is a past history of chromosomal abnormalities. Fetal sexing is important when dealing with X-linked inherited conditions. DNA analysis can also be carried out on the trophoblast cells and gene probes employed to detect inborn errors of metabolism, as well as diseases such as cystic fibrosis and Duchenne muscular dystrophy. Biochemical analysis using enzyme assays can also be used to detect certain inborn errors of metabolism.

Amniocentesis involves sampling amniotic fluid via a needle passed under ultrasound control through the abdominal wall into the amniotic cavity. There is a 1% risk of fetal loss as well as a small increased incidence of neonatal respiratory distress and postural deformities such as clubfoot. It is performed between 15 and 20 weeks depending on the indication. Reliable chromosome analysis can be performed on the amniotic cells which are derived from fetal skin, but this takes 2–3 weeks or more. Amniocentesis at 16 weeks is offered to all mothers over the age of 35 years (in some areas over 37) to exclude Down's syndrome. Most enzyme assays as well as DNA analysis can also be carried out on the amniotic cells.

Biochemical analysis can also be performed on the amniotic fluid. One of the main uses is to measure AFP levels to confirm the presence of a neural tube defect suspected after finding raised maternal serum AFP. Bilirubin levels in the second half of pregnancy give information on the severity of rhesus isoimmunization. Cystic fibrosis, congenital nephrotic syndrome and mucopolysaccharidoses can be diagnosed from products excreted into the fluid by the fetus.

Cordocentesis is a method of directly sampling fetal blood from the umbilical cord. It is carried out under ultrasound control in a similar way to amniocentesis. There is a 2% risk of fetal loss and a risk of fetomaternal haemorrhage. It can be used for fetal karyotyping and — as all cells are definitely of fetal origin, it can rule out a diagnosis of mosaicism which may have been indicated from amniocentesis or chorionic villous biopsy. Fetal blood is the principal way to diagnose some immunodeficiency disorders and α_1-antitrypsin deficiency biochemically, although these conditions can often be diagnosed using DNA markers. Cordocentesis is most useful, however, in haematological disorders. In rhesus incompatibility, fetal haemoglobin and haematocrit can be determined and if necessary the fetus can be given a blood transfusion. Haemoglobinopathies and coagulopathies can also be diagnosed.

Intrauterine growth retardation

The weight of the fetus can be estimated from measurements determined by ultrasound and compared to that expected for the gestational age. The gestational age is calculated from the date of the last menstrual period and is normally confirmed from the biparietal diameter measured at the routine 18-week scan. If an accurate estimate of gestational age has been made early in the pregnancy, then serial ultrasound measurements are a good indicator of fetal growth. Parameters measured include head circumference, abdominal girth, femur length and crown–rump length. Clinical examination is unreliable and will only detect the most severe cases, although oligohydramnios which often accompanies a small fetus may have been noted. Maternal weight gain in the last trimester may give guidance to IUGR. If the mother is otherwise well, and gains less than 0.5 kg/week for 3 weeks, inadequate fetal growth should be considered.

There are many causes of intrautererine growth retardation (IUGR) and these are dealt with in more detail on p. 121. There are two main categories: symmetrical and asymmetrical growth retardation. In the symmetrical type, the whole fetus is small with a normal ratio of head : abdominal circumference. These babies may simply be normal but small. However they also may have a chromosomal abnormality (e.g. Down's syndrome) or a major congenital abnormality (e.g. Potter's syndrome or anencephaly). The small size may also be associated with congenital infection, drugs, smoking and alcohol. It is important to exclude causes that can be reversed.

In asymmetrical growth retardation, the head seems to be spared at the expense of the rest of the body as the blood and nutrients preferentially go to the brain. Placental insufficiency is the main cause and may be associated with pre-eclampsia. These babies are at risk of ischaemic and hypoxic damage due to poor fetoplacental circulation, and this worsens during labour. Due to low levels of glycogen in the heart, these babies are also less able to tolerate asphyxia at birth. Their progress through pregnancy can be monitored by Doppler studies of blood flow through the uterine and umbilical arteries.

Despite intensive monitoring, IUGR is still associated with significant perinatal mortality and morbidity. No treatment improves fetoplacental insufficiency and delivery is usually the best option. The decision as to when to deliver the baby must take into account the associated risks of prematurity. After 28 weeks it is probably safest to go ahead with an elective Caesarean section.

Growth-retarded babies that have been stressed *in utero* tend to cope well in terms of respiratory problems but are at extra risk of hypothermia and hypoglycaemia (see p. 124). If the babies reach term, there is only a slightly increased risk of serious neurological impairment, but up to a third suffer from minor neurodevelopmental problems.

Fetal uropathies

Prenatal ultrasound examination detects many conditions that would be readily apparent at birth. However, one important role of scanning is diagnosis of fetal uropathies that would otherwise go undetected. Approximately one in 800 babies is born with a significant urological abnormality that has been diagnosed prenatally. We are not concerned here with those abnormalities that are lethal (e.g. renal agenesis) or so serious as to be immediately obvious. Some uropathies, such as vesico-ureteric reflux, may only become apparent later in childhood, manifest by urinary tract infections, but by then, renal scarring may have taken place. These abnormalities may be congenital and detectable *in utero* or at birth. The proportion that are detectable prenatally and the natural history of some of these conditions are not yet known.

Dilatation of the renal pelvis and the rest of the urinary tract is amenable to prenatal detection. Many of these cases spontaneously resolve later in the pregnancy. If dilatation is still present before birth, it is most important that these babies are identified on the postnatal ward. They should all have a renal ultrasound within the first 24–48 hours. If this is normal then a second scan should be performed at 4–6 weeks of age and if still normal, the child can be discharged from follow-up.

If the postnatal scan shows pelvi-calyceal dilatation, the child needs further investigation to exclude vesico-ureteric reflux, pelvi-ureteric junction obstruction or posterior urethral valves. This involves a micturating cystogram and then possibly a renal isotope scan after a few weeks. Antibiotic prophylaxis with trimethoprim (1–2 mg/kg at night) should be started until a definitive diagnosis has been made.

FURTHER READING

Chamberlain G (1992) *ABC of Antenatal Care*. British Medical Association, London.

De Swiet M (1989) *Medical Disorders in Obstetric Practice*. Blackwell Scientific Publications, Oxford.

Gibb D & Newell MR (1992) HIV infection in children. *Archives of Disease in Childhood*, **67**: 138–41.

James D (1990) Diagnosis and management of fetal growth retardation. *Archives of Disease in Childhood*, **65**: 390–4.

Thomas DFM & Gordon AC (1989) Management of prenatally diagnosed uropathies. *Archives of Disease in Childhood*, **64**: 58–63.

Whittle MJ & Connor JM (1989) *Prenatal Diagnosis in Obstetric Practice*. Blackwell Scientific Publications, Oxford.

3: Anticipating Problems —
During and After Delivery

DURING DELIVERY

The whole process of giving birth in hospital is geared towards monitoring fetal well-being and intervention should the fetus become distressed. The next chapter on 'Attending Deliveries' outlines many of the indicators of fetal distress and also discusses those deliveries in which a problem may be anticipated.

At delivery, certain unavoidable situations may arise which can lead to future problems. In anticipation of these problems, we have, in this chapter, outlined a protocol designed to minimize the adverse effects on the baby.

Birth asphyxia

Immediate resuscitation of an asphyxiated baby is discussed in Chapter 5. If the hypoxia was severe or prolonged there will probably be acute sequelae and, if anticipated, these may sometimes be prevented.

Indicators of severe hypoxia are:
- Apgar score <3 at 1 minute or <5 at 5 minutes;
- failure to establish spontaneous respiration by 15 minutes;
- no audible heartbeat at birth;
- cord blood or scalp pH <7.15.

Management is aimed at minimizing the effects of cerebral oedema and preventing convulsions. The baby should be admitted to a neonatal unit and the following should be monitored:
- Blood pressure, heart rate;
- urine output;
- arterial blood gas estimations;
- serum electrolyte levels, calcium and glucose.

Oxygen is given as required, but arterial Po_2 should be maintained at 8–12 kPa. Ventilation is only necessary if there are accompanying respiratory problems (Chapter 19).

No oral feeds should be given as there is often a paralytic ileus. Fluid intake should be restricted to 40 ml/kg/day for fullterm babies to counter the effect of inappropriate ADH secretion. Oliguria may indicate onset of acute renal failure due to renal ischaemia.

There is insufficient evidence that intracranial pressure is raised in the early stages after birth asphyxia. Therefore traditional manoeuvres to reduce intracranial pressure are not warranted. If anything, hyperventilating the baby to lower the arterial Pco_2 can be deleterious as a low Pco_2 can lead to cerebral vasoconstriction. This in turn reduces the availability of oxygen to the brain.

If there is a severe metabolic acidosis, i.e. pH < 7.15 and base excess > 10 mmol/l, this should be corrected with:
• albumin 20% IV (10–20 ml/kg) over 20 minutes,
• sodium bicarbonate IV over at least 30 minutes. The dose of bicarbonate in millimoles is calculated as follows:

$$\text{Base deficit (mmol/l)} \times \text{weight (kg)} \times 0.3$$

(1 mmol = 1 ml of 8.4% sodium bicarbonate). The sodium bicarbonate (8.4%) is so hyperosmolar that it should be diluted with 5% glucose solution in a ratio of 1 : 4 if it is being given directly into a vein. Alternatively it can be put into the burette containing the maintenance fluids.

Severe hypotension may be due to hypovolaemia so if the mean arterial pressure (MAP) falls below 30 mmHg, give:
• albumin 20% IV (10–20 ml/kg) over 20 minutes; *or*
• whole blood (20 ml/kg) over 60 minutes.
If there is no response to this volume expansion, the hypotension may be the result of myocardial ischaemia in which case extra colloid is inappropriate. A dopamine infusion may then be necessary.

Prophylactic anticonvulsants should be started and most neonatal units will have their own preferences. Here are some alternatives:
1 Phenytoin IV, loading dose of 15–20 mg/kg given over 20 minutes with maintenance dose of 8 mg/kg/day (this must be given undiluted because the drug precipitates if added to IV fluids).
2 Clonazepam IV, loading dose of 0.25 mg stat then infusion of

0.01–0.05 mg/kg/hour, titrating the dose according to the response.

3 Phenobarbitone IV or IM, loading dose of 15–20 mg/kg with maintenance dose of 5–10 mg/kg/day.

Poor neurodevelopmental prognosis is indicated by abnormal neurological signs that do not improve within a week. These include a lack of spontaneous limb movements, abnormal muscle tone (initially hypotonia followed by hypertonia) and absent primitive reflexes (see Appendix 3). One of the most significant signs is a failure to suck and swallow with an absent gag reflex. True assessment can not be carried out until the effects of sedative anticonvulsants have worn off.

Convulsions that last more than 48 hours are also a poor sign. In addition, if the convulsions start within the first hour, it implies the asphyxia was prolonged and not simply an acute episode just before birth.

Long-term follow-up is required before the nature of any handicap is made apparent. This may range from mild clumsiness to severe mental retardation with a spastic quadraplegia. Birth asphyxia may be superimposed on an underlying abnormality, which may have contributed to the cause of the abnormal labour. Only 10% of cerebral palsy is now considered to be related to events at birth.

Prolonged rupture of membranes

If the membranes are ruptured for over 24 hours, there is a risk of the baby becoming infected from contaminated liquor. Infection is particularly associated with repeated pelvic examinations.

The risk that the baby has been infected can be assessed at birth by performing a gastric aspirate. This should be done immediately after delivery and must be performed before the first feed. A nasogastric tube is passed and the stomach contents aspirated into a sterile syringe. The interpretation of gastric aspirates is controversial but the following is a scheme that can be used as a guide to the risk of infection.

A positive gastric aspirate is the presence of >5 polymorphonuclear cells per high-power field on microscopy. The presence of bacterial organisms has never been proved to be of any significance. Risk of infection is calculated from a points scheme:

1 point   gestational age <37 weeks,
1 point   maternal temperature during labour >38°C,
2 points   PROM >24 hours,
2 points   Apgar score <7 at 1 minute.

If the score is <2 i.e. no risk factors apart from prolonged rupture of membranes, there is minimal risk of infection, even if the gastric aspirate is positive. These babies need no active management apart from routine observation on the postnatal ward.

If the score is 3–4 points, there is a 5% risk. Blood cultures should be taken and the child observed on the ward. If the aspirate is positive, the risk of infection is doubled to 10% and these babies should receive IV antibiotics as well.

When the score is 5–6 points, the infection risk is high. It is 30% if the aspirate is negative and 40% if positive. These children must have blood cultures taken and immediately start IV antibiotics.

The most common pathogen is group B streptococcal infection which can cause rapidly progressive septicaemia or pneumonia (see p. 189). Benzylpenicillin is therefore the antibiotic of choice. If the blood cultures are negative after 48 hours, and the child remains well, antibiotics can be discontinued. If the mother has received more than one dose of antibiotic during labour, the blood cultures are irrelevant if negative. In this case, antibiotics must be given to the baby for 7 days.

At all times, clinical evidence of infection is paramount and should overrule this scheme. Pointers are pyrexia, tachypnoea, hypoglycaemia, irritability or poor feeding.

AFTER DELIVERY

Early identification of risk factors and illness in the newborn forms the major part of this book (Part 3). There are, however, certain aspects of the mother's behaviour on the postnatal ward which would give cause for concern. These may be noticed by an astute midwife or doctor and early intervention may help the mother.

Mother–infant attachment

There is a fundamental biological need for close mother–infant attachment. This gives the infant the degree of security necessary for optimal emotional and physical development. Whilst some mothers have strong maternal feelings that allow instant bonding with the baby, others find it difficult. The ability to bond is often related to the mother's own childhood experiences. Failure to form a normal attachment is a risk factor for subsequent child abuse.

There are certain pointers that may suggest that a particular mother is likely to have difficulty forming attachment to her baby.

Early separation is undesirable for all mothers, but the effect may be profound on those who are encountering difficulties with bonding in the first place. Separation is sometimes unavoidable. The baby may have to be transferred to another hospital for urgent surgery or may have to be sent to a neonatal unit if premature.

Drugs. The mother may be unwell herself, receiving heavy sedation for hypertension. Sometimes mothers feel distant after a general anaesthetic given for a Caesarean section.

Social problems. There are many examples of mothers who are particularly vulnerable. A mother may have requested an abortion which has been rejected. She may be an unmarried mother who has not decided whether she wishes the infant to be adopted, or she may be very young and under pressure from her own parents to have the baby adopted. The child may even be the result of rape.

Past history. A previous baby may have been stillborn or died in the neonatal period and this may lead to difficulties with bonding and extra anxiety (see p. 11).

Postnatal depression is often not obvious. Early signs may be a refusal to handle or feed the baby and the mother may be more concerned with her own minor symptoms than the infant's care.

The types of depression range in severity. The commonest form is the 'baby blues' seen after 3–4 days in over half the mothers. The women are weepy and feel despondent and anxious. It soon passes and all that is needed is understanding and reassurance. In addition to the psychological stresses of pregnancy and childbirth, the enormous hormonal changes following delivery play a part. Finally, in some cultures, the mother feels very guilty for having a baby girl instead of a boy.

True postnatal depression has an incidence of about 10%. It tends to manifest itself after 2 weeks and has all the features of a reactive depression (anxiety, irritability, insomnia, poor appetite, loss of libido). Professional help is usually needed in the form of psychotherapy or antidepressants. Practical help looking after the baby is also essential. Unfortunately there are appreciable difficulties in the mother–infant relationship for many months, and the emotional and cognitive development of the infant may be adversely affected.

Puerperal psychosis is fortunately uncommon. It manifests as a florid psychosis with hallucinations, delusions, confusion and sometimes mania. Nearly half the cases begin within a week of delivery and the rest appear over the next 3 months. There is a real risk of suicide or infanticide and the mother needs urgent admission to a mother and baby unit in a psychiatric hospital.

Abnormal babies may provoke ambivalent feelings in the mother, especially if she is already feeling guilty. It may be difficult for parents to bond with babies who are deformed, particularly if there are severe craniofacial abnormalities. Fortunately this does not tend to happen very often. If the baby is very ill or very premature, some parents try to distance themselves and not get too attached to the baby as a form of self-protection in case the baby dies.

The key to management of these problems is prevention and early recognition. Unnecessary separation must be avoided. The babies should be kept on the postnatal wards with their mothers if at all possible. Babies who require phototherapy, nasogastric feeling or even intravenous antibiotics should stay with their mothers.

When a baby is taken from the labour ward to the neonatal unit, instant photographs should be taken on arrival and sent down to the mother who may be detained in the delivery room.

If the child is transferred to another hospital, the parents should accompany him and facilities provided for the mother to stay. Mothers must have open access to their babies on neonatal units and be made to feel welcome. They can help with routine management such as changing nappies and feeding. They can also express breastmilk that can be given to the baby down a nasogastric tube if necessary. This will make them feel they are contributing to the welfare of their baby. They should also be encouraged to touch and talk to their babies. The needs of the fathers as well as older siblings and grandparents must also not be forgotten.

Once the mother has been discharged from hospital, she may need financial and practical help in order to visit every day. Before the baby is discharged from hospital, the mother should stay with the baby in a room on the unit for at least one night. This allows her to gain confidence in her ability to cope with her baby who until now has had full-time expert nursing care.

Part 2
The Labour Ward

4: Attending Deliveries

Paediatricians are frequently asked to be present during the delivery of a baby which can be very stressful for inexperienced doctors.

WHEN TO ATTEND

Most obstetric units have their own guidelines on when to call a paediatrician but these are the usual indications:

1 Fetal distress.
2 Meconium-stained liquor.
3 Caesarean section (elective and emergency).
4 Instrumental deliveries (e.g. forceps or ventouse suction extraction).
5 Narcotic analgesia administered to mother within 4 hours.
6 Breech presentations.
7 Premature and other small babies.
8 Twins and other multiple births.
9 Antenatally diagnosed abnormalities of the fetus.
10 Requests by the midwife or obstetrician for any other reason.

These high-risk deliveries account for two-thirds of babies requiring resuscitation, the remainder arise unexpectedly.

WHAT TO EXPECT

Fetal distress is the most worrying situation in which a paediatrician is called. This may have been suggested by abnormalities on the cardiotocograph, meconium-stained liquor, acidosis in fetal scalp capillary sample, an antepartum haemorrhage or a cord prolapse. In cases which require an emergency Caesarean section, nearly half the babies have an Apgar score (see Table 4.1) which indicates that intervention is required. However, if a spontaneous vaginal delivery is possible, only 10% have an Apgar score below 7 at 1 minute. Fortunately the majority of babies are born in excellent condition despite warning signals, but it is still a relief to hear that first cry.

Table 4.1 Assessing the Apgar score.

Factors to assess	Score		
	0	1	2
Heart rate	Nil	<100	>100
Respiratory effort	Absent	Gasping or irregular	Regular respiration or strong cry
Muscle tone	Limp	Reduced	Normal active movement
Response to stimulation	None	Grimace	Cry or cough
Colour of trunk	White	Blue	Pink

The parameters can be arranged into a useful mnemonic:

A ppearance: colour of trunk
P ulse: heart rate
G rimace: response to stimulation
A ctivity: muscle tone
R espiration: respiratory effort.

Meconium-stained liquor may be an indication of severe fetal distress particularly if it is fresh, thick and copious. Light staining, however, especially if it has occurred several hours previously is of little significance and unlikely to cause any problems. Management of 'meconium deliveries' can be difficult and is outlined on p. 68.

The outcome of a Caesarean section largely depends on the indication. Even elective sections can cause problems as the baby often arrives in a rather 'sleepy' condition and needs some stimulation to start breathing. Inexperienced paediatricians are often reassured by the presence of the anaesthetist but remember his or her prime duty is to the mother and unless there are two anaesthetists he or she will be unable to assist you.

In a similar way, the outcome of instrumental deliveries also depends on the indication. If forceps are used for a simple 'lift-out' then no problems should be anticipated, but rotational forceps (e.g. Kielland forceps) are a different matter and the baby often needs attention.

If the mother has received a narcotic analgesia such as pethidine within 4 hours of delivery, the baby may have respiratory depression and may need to be given an antagonist (see p. 67).

Breech presentations carry an increased risk to the baby particularly if delivered vaginally. The main problem is the potential for asphyxia when the trunk is delivered; the cord may be compressed while the head is still inside the pelvis. In addition, the baby may suffer trauma during extrication of the limbs and head.

The main problem at delivery of premature babies is lack of respiratory effort, particularly when less than 28 weeks gestation. They are extremely fragile and are also more prone to the effects of hypothermia.

Multiple births also give rise to more complications and ideally there should be one paediatrician present for each baby, particularly if the babies are also premature.

Antenatally-diagnosed fetal abnormalities such as severe hydrocephalus or anencephaly may be life-threatening. No active intervention may be possible but an experienced paediatrician should still be present.

WHAT TO DO

When you enter the delivery room introduce yourself immediately to the parents-to-be and explain what you are likely to do. Do not, however, start talking to them during one of the mother's contractions. You should wash your hands and it is advisable to wear gloves. Before you leave, do not forget to write in the notes even if you have not intervened; if there have been any complications then ensure that your notes are particularly clear and complete.

Establish the nature of the problem and get as much information as possible from the midwife. If there is time then read the obstetric notes. You should always check that the Resuscitaire is working and that you have all the necessary equipment and drugs you might need. More details of these are given in Chapter 5. It is useful to have your own set routine and reassuring to know that everything is in the same place on the Resuscitaire whenever you are at a difficult delivery.

When the baby is born the first thing to do is to assess whether any intervention is necessary. Most babies start to breathe after 10 seconds and if the baby cries instantly, then clearly you are not needed (except in cases of prematurity or fetal abnormality). The midwife can hand the baby immediately to the parents. Do not interfere with the baby just because you are there, simply offer your congratulations, write up the notes and leave. You should, however, wait 10 minutes before leaving after a Caesarean section as there may be delayed apnoea.

Routine care of the newborn will be carried out by the midwife. The forceps used on the umbilical cord when it is cut are replaced by a sterile disposable cord clamp. In most hospitals, vitamin K is given to all babies as prophylaxis against haemorrhagic disease of the newborn. It is usually given as an intramuscular injection but can be given orally. The dose is 1 mg for fullterm babies and 0.5 mg for premature babies. Finally, the baby is dried, wrapped in a warm blanket and given to the parents.

A more formal way of assessing the condition of the baby is always carried out and recorded by either the midwife or paediatrician. This is the Apgar score. In theory, assessment is performed at 1 and 5 minutes, but in practice it tends to be done retrospectively. If the baby has needed resuscitation then scores should be given for 1, 3, 5 and 10 minutes and even longer if necessary. Table 4.1 shows how the Apgar score is obtained.

5: Resuscitation of the Newborn

GETTING READY

While waiting for the baby to arrive, set up the Resuscitaire. Check it is working and that you have everything you might need.

1 *Overhead heater.* Turn it on.

2 *Oxygen.* Ensure the cylinder is turned on and that it is not empty. If the Resuscitaire runs off the wall supply then check it is connected. Oxygen flow rate should be set at 5 l/min. There is a second oxygen outlet which can be used to administer intermittent positive pressure ventilation when connected directly to the endotracheal tube. The blow-off valve should be permanently set so that the maximum pressure obtainable is 30 cmH$_2$O and this must be checked.

3 *Suction.* Check this is turned on and producing adequate pressure. Make sure that there is a catheter connected (size FG 8).

4 *Stethoscope.* Preferably paediatric size.

5 *Clock.* There should be a stop-clock that works.

6 *Tray.* The mattress on which the baby is placed is on an adjustable tray. This tray should be flat rather than tilted at an angle. Traditionally, it was kept at a slope to aid drainage of fluid from the pharynx, but the head-down position causes problems for the baby. It produces increased venous pressure in the brain leading to raised intracranial pressure. In addition, gravity ensures the intestines are pressed up against the diaphragm which makes it harder for the baby to breathe. Finally, the baby tends to slide down and is at risk of falling off the Resuscitaire.

7 *Face mask.* Soft funnel-shaped mask used for administering facial oxygen.

8 *Bag and mask.* A soft rubber self-inflating bag with a blow-off pressure valve which attaches to a round soft clear mask is the best system (e.g. Laerdal). Ensure the correct size mask is fitted — 2 or 1 for fullterm and 0 or 00 for preterm. Connect this to the oxygen supply and check it works. Put the mask against your hand so that a tight seal is formed. Then squeeze the bag and listen to the click made by the blow-off valve. This click will not be heard when there is an inadequate seal produced by the mask or if there is a leak in the system.

9 *Laryngoscope.* The small straight-blade should be fitted as it is the easiest one to use in babies. Open it out to check it works and that the bulb is bright enough. It is wise to have a spare laryngoscope which works available.

10 *Endotracheal tube (ETT).* Use the oral shouldered Cole blueline neonatal tubes (Portex) rather than nasal tubes which are difficult to use in an emergency. Size 3.0 mm for fullterm and 2.5 mm for preterm babies. The ETT comes with a blue endotracheal adaptor that fits the Laerdal bag and ventilator outlets. An introducer (stylet) can be used and it should be curved to the shape of the ETT. However, ensure the connector end of the stylet is kinked over so that the tip can not protrude through the end of the ETT otherwise it can perforate the airway. A connecting device should be available to attach the ETT to the baby in case it needs to be held in place for any length of time or adhesive tape can be used.

11 *Drugs.* The following should be available:

Adrenaline 1 in 10 000
Calcium gluconate 10%
Atropine
Sodium bicarbonate 8.4%
Glucose 10%
Naloxone HCl (Neonatal Narcan)
Vitamin K
Normal saline
Water for injection.

12 *BM Test 1–44.* BM stix must be available for estimation of blood glucose.

13 *Warm towels.* These should stay in the warming cabinet until the last moment.

Initial assessment

As soon as the baby is born, start the clock. The first assessment takes place even as the cord is being cut since the baby should cry once exposed to cold air. If there is an immediate yell and he continues to cry this indicates all is well. There is no need to interfere so do not take the baby over to the Resuscitaire automatically but give him to the parents. If he does not cry initially, then the midwife will bring him over to you.

Warming the baby

The first thing to do is to dry the baby then remove the wet towels that he is lying on and wrap him in a warm blanket. Put a hat on him as well. Keeping the baby warm is extremely important as hypothermia exacerbates acidosis and increases the baby's oxygen requirement. Wet asphyxiated babies rapidly become cold and low body temperature correlates with a poor prognosis.

At the same time, this process of rubbing him dry serves as good tactile stimulation and is preferable to slapping him on the feet. Be gentle as you can easily cause bruising which leads to jaundice, especially in premature babies.

Reassessment and initial treatment
Assessment is a continual process as the baby's condition can change rapidly. Although the Apgar scoring system is useful retrospectively for documenting progress, an overall impression of the baby is what will determine the course of action. A baby tends to fit into one of the following groups:
1 Vigorous and crying.
2 Gasping and bradycardic.
3 Pale, apnoeic and bradycardic.
4 Asystolic but potentially revivable.
5 Stillborn or macerated.

The baby is now reassessed in order to decide which of the following is necessary:
1 No further action.
2 Suction only.
3 Facial oxygen.
4 Bag and mask.
5 Intubation.
6 External cardiac massage.

No further action
If the baby is now crying with a good heart rate then resuscitation is no longer required. The normal procedures of clamping the cord and administering vitamin K are carried out and the baby returned to his parents who can then be reassured that all is well.

Sometimes resuscitation is inappropriate; see p. 69 for details.

Suction only
The baby may have large amounts of secretions or bloody liquor in the mouth and pharynx. If this is the case then gentle oropharyngeal suction should be performed. It also acts as a

stimulant but should not be used for this purpose. In an apnoeic baby, overzealous suctioning should not delay the onset of proper resuscitation. If the baby is breathing well with only a small amount of secretions present then leave him alone as the fluid will soon be swallowed or drain out. Suctioning is not without its complications; a suction tube applied to the posterior pharynx may cause apnoea so it must not be carried out unnecessarily.

Facial oxygen
The baby may be breathing spontaneously with a normal heart rate but remain mildly cyanosed. In this case you should administer oxygen via a face mask. After a few minutes the baby should be pink (apart from hands and feet) and the oxygen can be discontinued.

Bag and mask
If the baby is gasping or taking shallow irregular breaths and is bradycardic, then oxygen is administered using the bag and mask. The heart rate need not be counted as listening alone is sufficient to differentiate the normal fast rate of 120–160 from a bradycardic rate of 60 or less. Initially it is much safer to use the bag and mask than to intubate, particularly if you are inexperienced at intubation. Resuscitation with the bag and mask is successful in the majority of babies. The primary mechanism is not ventilation of the lungs but initiation of spontaneous breathing due to Head's paradoxical reflex. Rapid inflation of the lungs causes the baby to take an inspiration which is followed by gasps and then normal breathing.

Intubation
When the baby is in obvious terminal apnoea, immediate intubation with intermittent positive pressure ventilation (IPPV) is necessary. The baby appears pale or even white, is completely limp, makes no efforts at all to breathe and has bradycardia or asystole. In this situation there is no point in using the bag and mask first and you must intubate without delay. Fortunately this is an uncommon occurrence.

    You should have a lower threshold for intubating premature

babies. Those under 32 weeks gestation who are not breathing well should be intubated quickly and most babies under 28 weeks should be intubated electively for transfer to the neonatal unit.

External cardiac massage
Although rare, occasionally no heart beat is heard. Assuming the fetal heart beat had been detected prior to birth, then while the baby is being intubated someone must start external cardiac massage (ECM) and full cardiac arrest procedures are initiated.

PROGRESS

Once normal respiration is established and the baby has a normal heart rate, artificial ventilation can cease. If the bag and mask was being used then continue facial oxygen for a further few minutes. If bagging was necessary for a prolonged period, pass a nasogastric tube and aspirate the air that will have accumulated in the stomach.

If the baby has been intubated then once he is no longer bradycardic and is a good colour it is time to consider extubation. You may have already noticed the baby making initial gasps. With the ETT still in place stop the artificial ventilation for about 15 seconds and see if he breathes spontaneously. Although more difficult, the baby will be able to breathe through the ETT and it will soon be obvious if he is ready for extubation, particularly as he will try to reject the tube. Take it out and administer some facial oxygen for a short while. Occasionally the baby requires re-intubation but this is unusual.

LACK OF PROGRESS

If resuscitation is not succeeding, then move up a stage. If you are just administering facial oxygen then ventilate with the bag and mask. If this does not help then you must intubate the baby. Once intubated, the baby should improve rapidly and failure to do so is easy to recognize. The baby remains:
• white or blue;
• bradycardic;
• apnoeic or gasping.

In this case, you must quickly determine what is going wrong and immediately call for help from a more senior paediatric colleague. You must decide:

1 Is the baby intubated properly?
2 Is the oxygen getting to the baby?
3 Is external cardiac massage needed?
4 Should drugs be used?
5 Is there something else wrong with the baby?

Is the baby intubated properly?
It is easy to insert the endotracheal tube incorrectly during an emergency intubation and also common for it to become dislodged. It can end up in the oesophagus or go down too far, usually into the right main bronchus. The commonest signs that the ETT is not in the trachea are that the baby does not 'pink-up' and remains bradycardic. Additional indicators of misplacement are:
• lack of any chest movement;
• unequal chest movement (when in the right main bronchus);
• abdominal distension (stomach fills with air if it is in the oesophagus);
• crying sounds are heard (if the tube is correctly through the vocal cords the baby can not cry).
Listening with a stethoscope can be misleading, particularly in small babies, as breath sounds are easily transmitted to the lungs even if the ETT is in the oesophagus.

The ETT may have become blocked with thick secretions which are not always removed by a suction catheter so the tube should be changed. Check also that the ETT is not kinked.

The golden rule is: if in doubt, re-intubate.

Is the oxygen getting to the baby?
Check the oxygen is turned on and that the cylinder is not empty. Also make sure the supply has not become disconnected from the Resuscitaire and that the green oxygen tubing is connected properly.

Is external cardiac massage needed?
ECM will have already been started if no heart beat was detected

at birth. However, in a bradycardic baby if the heart rate falls below 40/minute or the pulses are weak, then cardiac output will be inadequate and you should begin ECM.

Should drugs be used?
If a baby requires ventilation and cardiac massage then you should also administer the emergency drugs. Adrenaline, particularly placed down the endotracheal tube, sometimes leads to a dramatic improvement. The use of drugs is a difficult area and is dealt with later in the chapter on p. 64.

Is there something else wrong with the baby?
If full resuscitative measures are still unsuccessful there may be an underlying reason and the following conditions should be considered: **1**, tension pneumothorax; **2**, pulmonary hypoplasia; **3**, prematurity; **4**, haemorrhage; **5**, diaphragmatic hernia; **6**, cardiac abnormalities.

1 *Tension pneumothorax.* This is a life-threatening emergency as the pleural cavity on the affected side of the chest expands with air. It causes the lung to collapse on the affected side, displaces the mediastinum to the opposite side and compresses the heart. Clues to the diagnosis are:

    (a) unilateral hyperexpansion of the chest,
    (b) lack of respiratory movement on the affected side,
    (c) shift of the apex beat to the opposite side.

Diagnosis can be confirmed with the use of a fibreoptic 'cold-light' source if this is available. When placed against the affected side it causes the whole hemithorax to glow brightly. There is no time for a chest X-ray.

If you suspect the diagnosis then the pleural cavity must be aspirated. Use a green 'butterfly' needle (size 21G) with the end held under water in a sterile bottle and put the needle into the chest (Fig. 5.1). It should go in 1–2 cm in the anterior-axillary line around the fourth and fifth intercostal space. If a pneumothroax is present the end in the water will bubble furiously and the baby's condition will rapidly improve. A proper chest drain will then have to be inserted. If there are no bubbles produced then there is no pneumothorax and the needle should be withdrawn.

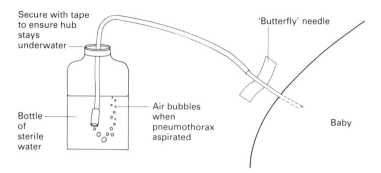

Fig. 5.1 Emergency aspiration of a tension pneumothorax.

2 *Pulmonary hypoplasia.* With pulmonary hypoplasia, the chest appears rather narrow. It is extremely difficult to ventilate these babies and the condition is usually fatal. It should be suspected if there has been oligohydramnios and is often associated with the rare Potter's syndrome and other postural deformities.

3 *Prematurity.* The baby may be more premature than realized although this should be obvious from the appearance. In this case there may be severe hyaline membrane disease and the lungs may require higher pressures to inflate them.

4 *Acute haemorrhage.* The baby may have lost a considerable amount of blood which can go unnoticed. This can be due to haemorrhage from the placenta or umbilical cord during delivery or an antepartum haemorrhage. It may also be due to a twin-to-twin transfusion. The baby appears extremely pale and may be tachycardic with a poor pulse volume. Immediate transfusion with 10–20 ml/kg uncrossmatched O-negative blood is required. Give the first 20 ml in 3 minutes. If blood is not immediately available use albumin to correct the hypovolaemia if the baby is shocked.

5 *Diaphragmatic herniae.* Diaphragmatic herniae are usually left-sided. The herniated stomach and bowel compress the lung and displace the mediastinum and heart to the opposite side. Poor air entry on the left, shift of the apex beat to the right, and a scaphoid abdomen are clues, but an X-ray is needed to confirm the diagnosis. If suspected, do not use the bag and mask as this causes gaseous distension of the bowel in the chest. You must intubate immediately and keep the stomach empty with a nasogastric tube.

6 *Cardiac abnormalities.* Congenital cardiac disease does not usually present as a resuscitation problem unless the lesion is extremely severe, in which case the infant is usually stillborn.

METHODS OF RESUSCITATION

Suctioning the oropharynx
It is best not to use mucus extractors as there is a risk of the operator swallowing or inhaling infectious material. Use a suction catheter (size FG 8) connected to the Resuscitaire or directly to a wall suction unit. The mouth can safely be suctioned but care must be taken in the oropharynx. This should be done under direct vision and is usually part of tracheal intubation. Do not blindly push the catheter as far as it will go since this can cause a vagally-mediated bradycardia and apnoea and is invariably associated with a drop in oxygen saturation.

Administering facial oxygen
Set the oxygen flow rate to 5 l/min and hold the funnel-shaped mask just in front of the baby's face. The oxygen may be connected either to the funnel-shaped mask or to the bag and mask apparatus, but in the case of the latter, it is prevented from flowing out of the mask by the valve unless the bag is compressed. However, it will come out of the corrugated tube which is attached to the other end of the bag so turn it round and hold the end of this tube to the baby's face (Fig. 5.2).

Using the bag and mask
The left hand is used to hold the mask to the baby's face while the right hand squeezes the bag. Place the little and ring fingers of your left hand under the baby's chin and with gentle traction slightly extend the neck. This prevents the head from moving around and straightens the upper airways, ensuring their patency. With the other fingers and thumb, apply the mask firmly to the baby's face to ensure a tight seal (Fig. 5.3). A proper seal is

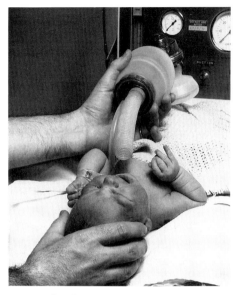

Fig. 5.2 Administering facial oxygen.

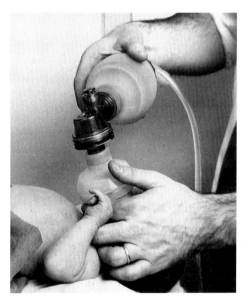

Fig. 5.3 Using the bag and mask.

confirmed when you squeeze the bag as there is a characteristic rasping noise as the valve opens. If the seal is inadequate, the valve makes no noise and you will not feel any resistance when squeezing the bag. This can be practised with the mask against the palm of your hand. Use only the thumb and two fingers, rather than your whole hand, to squeeze the bag. Do not empty the bag but gently depress it to a few centimetres only. This will safeguard against a pneumothorax. The smaller the baby, the gentler you must be. The rate should be maintained at 40/minute with an inflation time of approximately 1 second. Check you are producing an adequate chest expansion.

Intubation

Intubation is not difficult if you understand the anatomy (Figs 5.4 & 5.5). The easiest babies to intubate are those in poor condition as they lie still without gasping and the vocal cords remain apart. Indeed if a baby is struggling against you then intubation is probably unnecessary.

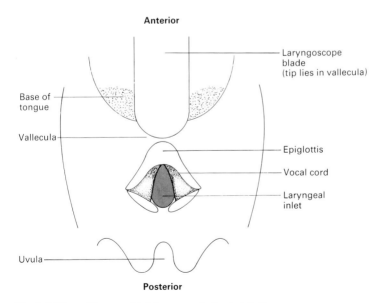

Fig. 5.4 View of laryngeal inlet as seen during intubation.

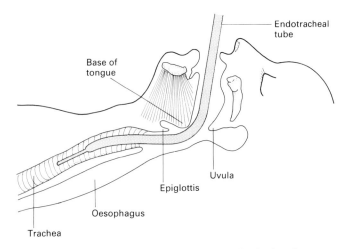

Fig. 5.5 Sagittal section to show position of endotracheal tube after intubation.

It is a delicate procedure and you must be gentle. The laryngoscope can traumatize the tissues, leading to bruising and oedema and can cause laryngospasm if used forcibly. It can also induce a vagally-mediated bradycardia and raise intracranial pressure. Remember also that during the intubation the infant is not getting any oxygen so if you are having difficulty you should stop after 20–30 seconds. Someone else can ventilate the baby with the bag and mask while you compose yourself for another attempt.

Position the baby so that he is lying straight with his head in the midline and neck slightly extended. Hyperextending the neck by placing something under the shoulders is unnecessary. Take the laryngoscope in your left hand. Do not hold the handle in the palm of your hand as this does not allow delicate movement. Hold it between your thumb and the tips of your index, middle and ring fingers (Figs 5.6 & 5.7). Before you can insert the endotracheal tube you must visualize the entrance to the larynx. It is a dark slit or triangular hole in the centre of a small pink mound. It is flanked by the two white vocal cords and anteriorly it is guarded by the epiglottis which is a shiny pink, leaf-like structure. Looking through the laryngeal opening you can see the tracheal rings as the trachea is a direct continuation of the lower part of the larynx.

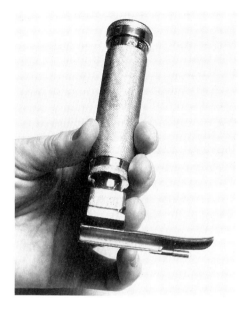

Fig. 5.6 Holding the laryngoscope.

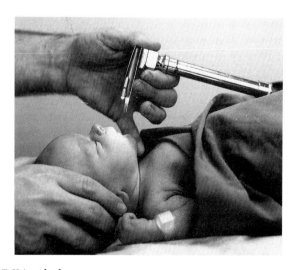

Fig. 5.7 Using the laryngoscope.

Lock open the blade and this lights the bulb. You may have to open the baby's mouth with your right hand. Gently slide the blade downwards and backwards over the top of the tongue. At this stage you do not usually see the vocal cords but may see the epiglottis. A common mistake is to push the blade down too far so if you see nothing withdraw it slightly. If you can not see the epiglottis then you need to apply 'cricoid pressure'. It is best to do this yourself and this is why the little finger of your left hand is free and not holding the laryngoscope. With the little finger, exert gentle downward pressure over the cricoid cartilage which is in the centre of the anterior part of the neck. You will now see the epiglottis but still may not see the vocal cords.

The tip of the blade should be above (i.e. anterior to) the epiglottis in the vallecula. The epiglottis may obscure the view of the cords but do not try to flick it upwards with the blade. Instead the cords can be brought into view by a gentle upward pressure (anteriorly) of the blade in the vallecula. This is achieved with a slight rotation at the wrist (pronation) as if drinking from a glass and is a very delicate movement. It has the effect of lifting the whole laryngeal inlet. It may be helpful to extend the neck a little further. The cords may be closed together (adducted) but will move apart as the baby gasps. In a completely apnoeic baby they are usually fully abducted allowing a good view of the target.

Everything may be obscured by thick mucus and the assistant should put the suction catheter into your right hand. Do not take your eyes off the laryngeal opening. Suction the area quickly and then the assistant can take the catheter from you and put the endotracheal tube in your right hand.

The rest is relatively easy. Slide the ETT down and pass it through the vocal cords 1–2 cm into the trachea. You may need to introduce the ETT from the corner of the mouth and it sometimes needs some manoeuvring to position it correctly. Just as the tube approaches the entrance to the larynx, it often obscures the view, particularly in small babies, so this very last part is done blindly. It is at this point, if you are not careful, that the tube slips too far posteriorly and into the oesophagus.

When the ETT is in the trachea, remove the laryngoscope. Hold the tube in place with the index finger of your left hand by pushing the tube up against the hard palate. It is easy at this stage for it to become dislodged if you do not hold it firmly. Remove the introducer if you used one and connect the ventilation bag to the ETT. Before fixing the tube, you must be sure it is in the correct place. Successful intubation is indicated by:

• chest movement synchronous with squeezing the bag;
• improvement in heart rate;
• improvement in the baby's colour;
• improvement in oxygen saturation (if monitor is available).

Listening to breath sounds is useful to check that both lungs are being equally ventilated (i.e. ETT is not in the right main bronchus) but should not be used to indicate that the ETT is in the trachea. If you suspect it is down too far withdraw it slowly 0.5–1 cm while still listening.

It is safer to ventilate an intubated baby with the inflatable bag rather than directly off the Resuscitaire. It is more sensitive and there is less chance of causing a pneumothorax. However compression of the bag must be even more gentle than when using it with the mask as the air pressure is directly transmitted to the lungs. Respiratory rate should be maintained at 40/minute allowing 1 second for inflation. The very first inflation should be held for 2–3 seconds to expand the lungs fully. If you use the Resuscitaire for IPPV and the baby has not yet gasped, you need an initial inflation pressure of 30 cmH$_2$O to open up the alveoli. Pressures of higher than 30 cmH$_2$O are occasionally needed initially but are more hazardous and can only be provided by the inflatable bag. After a short while, you can reduce the pressure to 10–20 cmH$_2$O depending on the stiffness of the lungs.

If intubation is to be continued, then you need to decrease the dead space by cutting off the last 1–2 cm of the ETT. Note which size ETT was used, and check how far down it goes from the mouth by reading the centimetre marks on the side of the tube (it should be 8–9 cm in a fullterm baby). Pass a nasogastric tube and empty the stomach contents to avoid the risk of aspiration. Finally, a chest X-ray to confirm its position is required if ventilation is to continue.

Giving mouth-to-mouth resuscitation
Should there be major equipment failure, while replacements are

found it is still necessary to ventilate the baby. This can be done with mouth-to-mouth or mouth-to-tube ventilation. If the baby is not intubated put in an oral airway and extend the neck. Your mouth should cover the baby's mouth and nose. Due to the disparity in lung size you should blow rather than fully exhale into the baby, empty your cheeks rather than your lungs of air. If available, put the oxygen tubing into your own mouth as this gives the baby extra oxygen.

Giving external cardiac massage
Be gentle as it is easy to rupture the liver or spleen in small babies. Encircle the baby's chest with both hands with your thumbs resting over the mid-sternum. Depress the sternum 1–2 cm at a rate of 100/minute. Compression time should be 50% of the total cycle, so allow equal time for compression and decompression of the sternum. The rhythm is four cardiac compressions for every lung inflation. This is the most efficient method in terms of cardiac output and blood pressure obtainable. The other method involves depressing the mid-sternum using your index and middle fingers, and although less efficient, this method may be convenient when there is limited space.

USE OF DRUGS

If the baby is still apnoeic despite intubation and ventilation or is requiring ECM for asystole or severe bradycardia, then drugs are necessary. They can be administered by the following routes:
1 *Intratracheal* (IT). Instilling drugs down the endotracheal tube is an excellent way of giving adrenaline and atropine. It can be used immediately and the lungs absorb drugs quickly. The dose is double the IV dose and you need to dilute the drugs first in 2 ml normal saline. Inject the drug down the ETT, and then recommence ventilation which ensures the drug reaches the lungs.
2 *Intravenous* (IV). In a collapsed baby it is almost impossible to insert a peripheral intravenous line and the peripheral circulation is so sluggish that drugs would be poorly absorbed. However, emergency central venous access can be obtained using an umbilical venous catheter (UVC).
   Clean the cord then cut through it with a scalpel blade. If the

artery spurts blood simply compress the whole cord between your fingers. There are two arteries and one vein. The vein is recognized as it is larger with a thin wall and has an irregular outline whereas the arteries are small round thick-walled vessels. Remove any clot that may be sitting in the opening of the vein. After flushing a PVC catheter (blueline umbilical cannula size 6 FG) with normal saline, insert it gently to about 5 cm and you should be able to withdraw blood. Make sure the blood does not pulsate as this means you have cannulated the artery. The line is kept in place by tying a linen ligature round the whole cord which is also used to tie off the cord once the UVC is removed. It can now be used to give drugs but remember to flush them with saline or the small volumes may not clear the end of the catheter. Give the drugs slowly, at least over 1 minute and be scrupulous about avoiding air bubbles.

3 *Intracardiac* (IC). This is extremely hazardous as it is easy to puncture the lung or rupture a coronary artery. Although traditionally used as a last resort when there is nothing to lose, there is little to gain if you already have central venous access. The drugs do not work any better just because they are in the heart so use this route only if you have no other venous access. The technique is to insert a green needle (21G) at the xiphisternal angle, aiming upward and posteriorly. Alternatively, insert it medial to and below the left nipple (fourth intercostal space) and aim for the spine. Suck back on the syringe as you advance the needle until blood is aspirated.

There is no standard protocol as to the order in which drugs should be given but here is one suggested scheme:

1 Adrenaline 1 in 10 000.
2 Repeat the adrenaline.
3 Sodium bicarbonate 8.4%.
4 Calcium gluconate 10%.
5 Glucose 10%.
6 Repeat sodium bicarbonate, adrenaline and calcium gluconate.
   Other drugs that may be required are:
• albumin 5%;
• atropine;
• naloxone HCl (Neonatal Narcan).

Table 5.1 shows the recommended doses.

Table 5.1 Recommended doses.

Drug	Concentration	Route	Dose (ml/kg)	Dose for 3kg baby (ml)
Adrenaline	1 in 10 000 (0.1 mg/ml)	IT*, IV, IC	0.1	0.3
Calcium gluconate	10%	IV	0.2	0.6
Sodium bicarbonate	8.4% (1 mmol/ml)	IV	1	3 (dilute 1 : 4 with water)
Glucose	10%	IV	1–2	3–6
Albumin	5%	IV	10–20	30–60
Atropine	600 µg/ml	IV, IT*	0.03	0.09
Naloxone HCl	20 µg/ml	IM, IV	0.5	1.5

* Double the dose for intratracheal route

Adrenaline
Adrenaline is given when there is no heartbeat or for persistent bradycardia. It produces an increase in heart rate and myocardial contractility leading to an increase in cardiac output, hence it improves myocardial and cerebral perfusion. The intratracheal route is safe, with a rapid onset and a more prolonged action than the intravenous route.

Calcium gluconate
Calcium is also used for persistent severe bradycardia and asystole. It acts as a cardiotonic drug increasing myocardial contractility and raising blood pressure. It should never be given by the intracardiac route as it may cause necrosis of the myocardium and arrhythmias. It must not be mixed with bicarbonate as this causes it to precipitate.

Sodium bicarbonate
Bicarbonate is given to correct the acidosis that inevitably accompanies hypoxia. However its use is not clear cut as initially it causes a paradoxical intracerebral acidosis, and it can decrease

oxygen delivery to tissues. Overall it is still worth giving as adrenaline does not work well in the presence of acidosis and the bicarbonate may make the crucial difference. Once ventilation is established (to blow off the extra CO_2 generated) it can be given slowly, over at least 10 minutes. Since it is so hyperosmolar it must be diluted 1:4 with water.

Glucose

Many asphxiated babies are hypoglycaemic, especially if growth-retarded, and this causes metabolic derangements in the myocardium and central nervous system. After its use, monitor the blood glucose to detect any hyperglycaemia or rebound hypoglycaemia. If the baby is hypoglycaemic and venous access is not available, give an intramuscular injection of 250 µg glucagon.

Albumin

Albumin is used as a plasma volume expander and helps correct metabolic acidaemia. If not available, crystalloid alternatives such as 0.9% sodium chloride solution, Ringer's lactate or Hartmann's solution can be used.

Atropine

Atropine may be useful for prolonged bradycardia particularly if vagally-mediated which is the case in asphyxia. It can be given intravenously or down the endotracheal tube. A potential problem is that bradycardia is the best guide to lack of success in resuscitation and if this response is abolished a false picture may be given.

Naloxone

Naloxone, which is an opiate antagonist, is indicated if the mother received a narcotic analgesia such as pethidine within 4 hours of delivery. It should not be given until ventilation has been established. It is best to use the intramuscular route as it has a more prolonged effect. Although the intravenous route works sooner, it does not last long and the dose may have to be repeated as the effects of pethidine may last several hours. If the first dose has not worked, it can be repeated after 2–3 minutes.

MECONIUM DELIVERIES

The passage of meconium is a sign of fetal distress and a warning that the baby may be in poor condition at birth. A secondary problem is that the baby may inhale meconium-stained liquor during delivery. This can cause the meconium-aspiration syndrome which results in severe ventilatory problems (see p. 210).

To avoid this, as soon as the head appears you must thoroughly suck out the mouth and oropharynx. When the baby is completely delivered, take him quickly to the Resuscitaire for further suctioning. 'Chest compression' has been recommended in the past whereby the midwife squeezes the chest immediately so that the baby is unable to take a first gasp until the oropharynx has been suctioned, but it is no longer recommended. In reality it hardly ever worked and the baby cried before reaching the Resuscitaire, hence it is best to start suction while the head is at the perineum.

If there is a large amount of meconium you need to directly visualize the vocal cords with the laryngoscope and suck away any meconium from around the laryngeal inlet. You may need to insert an endotracheal tube and suction meconium from the trachea. This is not easy as the babies tend to be large, slippery and struggling. It may help to repeatedly inject 0.5 ml saline down the ETT and suck it back immediately but this is only advisable if you are experienced. Alternatively, you can attach the suction directly to the ETT but then you need to keep changing the tube.

Babies who are covered in meconium will have swallowed some as well. Aspirate the stomach contents with a nasogastric tube otherwise they regurgitate mucus for days and feed poorly.

FOLLOW-UP

A baby who required only facial oxygen or ventilation with the bag and mask will have recovered quickly. Further problems are unlikely and the baby should go to the postnatal ward with the mother. Similarly, a baby that required intubation for a few minutes should suffer no sequelae and will not need further follow-up.

Babies that required more intensive or prolonged resuscitation will need to be cared for on a neonatal unit to minimize the effects of hypoxia, which include cerebral oedema and convulsions (see p. 36). These infants will also need long-term follow-up to assess neurological development. The survival rate of fullterm newborn infants who have taken 20 minutes to breathe spontaneously is about 50% and about 75% of the survivors are neurologically intact.

If a baby dies or is stillborn and there is no obvious cause, blood should be taken for chromosomal analysis. It can be aspirated from the heart in a similar way to that described for administering intracardiac drugs. Put 2 ml into a lithium heparin bottle and if necessary it can be stored overnight in a fridge.

When to stop
Poor outcome can be predicted when spontaneous respirations are not established by 30 minutes. If, in addition, there is no cardiac output then survival cannot be expected. It is at this stage that attempts at resuscitation should cease.

When not to start
This can be an extremely difficult decision and should not be made by the most junior paediatrician, so begin resuscitation and call for help. If the heart rate has been recorded at any time during the second stage of labour, resuscitation should be attempted even if there is no heartbeat at birth. With fetal monitoring it is uncommon for babies to die during labour and stillbirths are usually expected. Babies who have been dead for longer than 12 hours have an obvious 'macerated' appearance with gross peeling of the skin.

A baby born at less than 24 weeks gestation cannot survive and often a paediatrician will not be called if the obstetrician is sure of the dates. Certain conditions are non-viable such as anencephaly or gross hydrocephaly but fortunately these are usually detected prior to birth and a decision is reached with the parents before delivery.

Helping the parents
The responsibility of the paediatrician does not stop when a baby dies or is stillborn. The parents will need considerable help both

immediately and in the future. Parents should be encouraged to see and to hold the baby and may want to be left alone with him. Be patient, try to answer their questions and give them enough time. Photographs and other mementos such as name tags should be offered to them. A sensitive and considerate approach will help them through the early stages of grieving.

FURTHER READING

David R (1988) Neonatal resuscitation: historical perspective and current practice. In: Guthrie RD (ed) *Neonatal Intensive Care*, pp. 1–20 Churchill Livingstone, Edinburgh.

6: Birth Injuries

Despite trauma, which is unavoidable in some deliveries, birth injuries are rare. The injuries typically affect the presenting part of the baby, usually the head, but fortunately they are rarely serious.

HEAD

Caput succedaneum
A 'caput' is the soft tissue swelling which causes the elongated head often noted at birth. It is seen, to some degree, in almost every baby, being absent only in those born by elective Caesarean section or breech deliveries. The subcutaneous oedema is not limited by the sutures and can involve the eyelids. It affects the part of the head presenting at the cervix which is subject to trauma with every contraction of the uterus. It usually resolves after a few days. An equivalent swelling is sometimes seen in a limb or the buttocks when these are the presenting parts in a breech delivery.

Cephalhaematoma
This is a subperiosteal haemorrhage, which tends to occur in the

parietal region, and since it is limited by the surrounding sutures will not cross the midline. It is likely that in many cases there is an underlying hairline fracture of the skull but this is unimportant as it involves only the outer table. A surprisingly large amount of blood may be present and you should check the baby's haemoglobin level if the haematoma is extensive. A haemoglobin level of 12 g/dl or less in the first 2 days of life may be an indication for a blood transfusion. Onset of jaundice can be anticipated due to breakdown of the large clot. A cephalhaematoma may take up to 6 weeks to resolve and during this time a calcified rim may appear which falsely suggests a depressed fracture. Sometimes a hard swelling appears due to calcification of the whole haematoma which is present for several months.

'Chignon'
Vacuum extraction is often associated with a 'chignon' or subcutaneous oedema where the cap has been applied. In some instances this may become a large haematoma and occasionally the skin becomes necrotic. However, the skin grows rapidly from the borders to cover the area within a few weeks.

Traumatic cyanosis
Sometimes the whole face is badly bruised or congested and it can give a false impression of cyanosis. Petechiae on the head and neck are common and are not significant as long as the rest of the body is not involved. Resolution is seen within 2–3 days.

Subconjunctival haemorrhages
Tiny haemorrhages, similar to the head and neck petechiae of traumatic cyanosis, are often seen against the white sclerae. They soon fade and cause no problems.

Facial palsy
Direct pressure by obstetric forceps on the facial nerve may cause a transient palsy leading to a weakening of one side of the face. It can also occur without the use of forceps in which case the nerve will have been compressed against the mother's pelvic bone. Although it often lasts only a few hours, and usually resolves

spontaneously within 1–2 days, facial palsy may sometimes take several months to improve. If the eye will not close then care of the cornea is essential. This condition must be differentiated from an asymmetric crying facies (see p. 92).

Other lesions
A fetal scalp electrode or capillary blood sampling may leave a small abrasion on the head. When the abrasions are large, they must be differentiated from a congenital absence of part of the scalp (cutis aplasia). This abnormality usually occurs in the region of the 'crown' and is 2–3 cm diameter. Scarring and healing take place over several months. The advice of a plastic surgeon with careful documentation is essential to preclude later litigation.

Forceps marks are often seen on the face and soon disappear. Occasionally, subcutaneous fat necrosis occurs in the area of skin to which the forceps pressure was applied. This leads to firm red or purple lumps which resolve spontaneously by 4–6 weeks.

Rarely, tiny cuts caused by a scalpel blade during a Caesarean section are noticed on the head or other parts of the body. Steristrips are all that is usually needed, but occasionally one or two sutures are required.

SHOULDER

Fracture of the clavicle
This usually occurs during a difficult breech extraction or with a shoulder dystocia. It presents with lack of movement in the arm on the affected side, or sometimes the mother notices that the child cries when she moves his arm whilst changing his clothes. A 'step' may be felt in the clavicle and diagnosis is confirmed by an X-ray. No treatment is necessary but it must be documented as at a later date it could be misinterpreted as a previous non-accidental injury.

Fracture of the humerus
This presents in a similar way to a fractured clavicle. Occasionally the radial nerve is affected as it spirals round the upper humerus which may cause a transient wrist drop. The arm

should be splinted to the infant's chest by a crepe bandage for 2–3 weeks.

Brachial plexus injury

This is usually caused by over-stretching the neck to one side during a delivery when the shoulder has been difficult to deliver and is often accompanied by a fractured clavicle. Classically the upper roots are involved producing an Erb's palsy. This presents with lack of arm movement and the arm takes on the characteristic 'waiter's-tip' posture. The phrenic nerve may also be involved which paralyses the hemi-diaphragm and causes tachypnoea. Occasionally the lower roots of the plexus are affected causing paralysis of the small muscles of the hand and forearm. The plexus is usually compressed by a haematoma or the nerves are simply stretched rather than torn. This means full neurological recovery is to be expected but if there is still a palsy at 2 weeks then the prognosis should be less optimistic. Physiotherapy is necessary in order to avoid limb contractures.

NECK

Sternomastoid 'tumour'

This is not noticeable at birth but usually presents after the first week. The firm swelling, 1–2 cm in diameter, may be situated anywhere along the length of the sternomastoid muscle, but is usually in the middle or lower third. It is caused by a small haematoma or fibromatous malformation and the resultant shortening in the muscle may cause a torticollis with the head held towards the same side. The lump tends to have disappeared by 6 months but gentle physiotherapy will help stretch the muscle and prevent further contracture.

TESTES

Haematoma

Bruising of the scrotum or actual haematoma of the testis may be seen after an extended breech delivery, as the scrotum may be the presenting part. No treatment is necessary and it resolves spontaneously within 1–3 weeks.

Part 3
The Postnatal Ward

7: Routine Examination of the Newborn

Immediately after birth, all babies are examined by the midwife, and undoubtedly scrutinized by both parents. Major abnormalities will be noticed at this stage and the paediatrician contacted. All babies should, however, be examined again in more detail by the paediatric house officer, preferably within 24 hours although the baby should be at least 6 hours old. With the present trend of early discharge this may be the only time the child is seen by a paediatrician.

The main object of this examination is to screen for hidden abnormalities such as congenital dislocation of the hip or heart disease, but it also reassures parents about minor abnormalities and normal variants. Thus although very routine for the doctor, this examination is very important for the parents who often wait anxiously for their baby to be 'passed' by the paediatrician. The mother should always be present so that she can ask any questions and express any concerns. This is particularly so if this is her first baby as what may seem trivial to you may be causing great alarm to the parents.

Be considerate and do not wake a baby who has finally fallen asleep after several fractious hours. Ideally, the examination should take place when the baby is alert and calm but if this is not possible then the next best time is when he is sleepy soon after a feed. Although it is hard to neurologically assess a sleeping baby, it is practically impossible to do anything at all if he is hungry and screaming. If he wakes after a feed he will soon go back to sleep but be careful not to make the baby vomit if he has a full stomach.

Wash your hands and warm them before seeing each baby. Finally, do not refer to the baby as 'it' or by the wrong gender.

HISTORY

Read the obstetric notes with particular attention to the following:
1 Problems during pregnancy such as polyhydramnios, infections or abnormal antenatal ultrasound examinations.

2 Expected date of delivery.
3 Labour and delivery (e.g. length, mode, complications).
4 Maternal medical and drug history.
5 Family history with emphasis on other siblings.
6 Social problems such as unsupported mother or drug abuse.

This will highlight problems and the parents' worries can be more readily understood. Some of these issues have already been discussed in Chapters 1 and 2.

DISCUSSION WITH MOTHER

Always introduce yourself and explain what you have come to do, then find out if she has any particular concerns. Check how the mother is and be alert if she seems overtired or depressed. Ask her how she is feeding the child and whether this is going well. Make sure you do not patronize new mothers or undermine their confidence.

CHARTS

Do not forget to look at the charts at the end of the bed. They will tell you about the temperature, pulse and respiratory rate of the baby. Weight changes and feeding patterns are also recorded as well as any blood glucose tests (BM stix) which may have been done. Time and date of delivery as well as birthweight, length and head circumference will be found on the blue or pink card attached to the cot but should also be recorded in the notes.

PHYSICAL EXAMINATION

This should be done systematically to avoid missing anything, proceeding from head to foot, but like all paediatric examinations you need to take advantage of opportunities. If the baby is crying then look in the mouth, if he opens his eyes then take advantage as you may not get a second chance. The baby should be completely undressed in a warm room, but remove the nappy at the last minute to avoid a shower with urine.

With experience, you will develop your own systematic approach but here is one suggested scheme:

1 General appearance.
2 Listen to the heart and lungs.
3 Head and neck.
4 Chest.
5 Abdomen.
6 Anus and genitalia.
7 Femoral pulses.
8 Limbs.
9 The back.
10 Hips.
11 Head circumference.

Before going any further, it is worth outlining how to pick up and hold a baby. Although they should be handled gently, babies are in fact rather robust. The head should be supported in the palm of your left hand with the fingers and thumb curled round. The baby's back rests on the flattened right hand with the rest of the weight supported by your right forearm. As a precaution, it is wise to encircle the baby's upper left arm in your right thumb and index finger, then if the baby slips you can instantly grip the arm tightly (see Fig. 7.1).

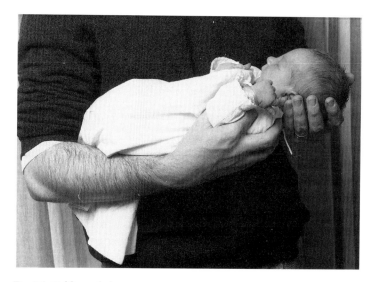

Fig. 7.1 Holding a baby.

General appearance

Dysmorphism. Gross structural abnormalities will have been noticed at birth, particularly if there is an abnormal facies, but the appearance may be more subtle. If there are a number of odd features then an expert opinion from a clinical geneticist may be necessary. A word of warning though, funny-looking children often have funny-looking parents so look carefully in case it is simply a family trait.

Colour. Good light — preferably natural — is necessary to assess a baby's colour. Confusion can be caused by reflection off bedspreads or bedside curtains. Pale babies may be anaemic or simply have very fair skin. Dark red babies are probably polycythaemic (see p. 176). Yellow babies have jaundice and this needs follow-up, particularly if it appears in the first 24 hours (Chapter 15). 'Blue babies' with cyanosis often appear light grey rather than blue and obviously this is a very serious sign if it is central (see p. 217). Cyanosis of the hands and feet, however, is a normal finding in the first 48 hours and is known as acrocyanosis, but after this time it is a non-specific but important sign of illness. Babies who are green have been stained with meconium and need a bath. These colour changes are more difficult to assess in racially pigmented babies but the palms of the hands, soles of the feet, or gums may be helpful if there is doubt about the colour of the skin.

Skin. Newborn babies have extremely smooth skin. However, if they are premature then it is thin and gelatinous, whereas if they are postmature it becomes dry and cracked and tends to peel, sometimes taking weeks to appear normal. Immediately after birth many babies are covered in a greasy cheese-like white material (vernix caseosa) found particularly in the folds of the neck and groin, which disappears within hours. Minor skin abnormalities and blemishes are very common and will be outlined in Chapter 8.

Posture and movements. A normal term baby lies with strongly flexed hips, knees and elbows. Children born with an extended breech (hips flexed, knees extended) tend to lie with their feet up by their ears for the first few days. Babies move their limbs and wriggle around spontaneously, they even stretch and yawn.

Crying. The normal cry, however piercing, must be differentiated from an abnormally high-pitched cry which may denote a neurological abnormality. A weak and feeble cry may also indicate that something is amiss.

Listen to the heart and lungs

It is best to do this early on if the baby is still quiet. If he is already crying then try stroking his cheek by the side of the mouth and let him suck your finger. This is the rooting reflex and is nearly always successful in calming the baby for several minutes before he realizes that no milk is coming. In the meanwhile you can be listening to the chest. It is better to use a paediatric or neonatal size stethoscope which should not be cold.

Listen over the heart areas with one question in mind. Is there a murmur present? The neonatal heart is beating so fast (110–160 times/minute) that you are not expected to detect minutiae but you should be able to hear a systolic murmur even if it is soft. These are extremely common in the first 48 hours of life and are dealt with on p. 227.

Next listen to the breath sounds which should be equal on both sides and clear. Faint crepitations may be heard in the first hours of life, usually due to retained fetal lung fluid which will be absorbed spontaneously. Coarse sounds are often heard caused by loose secretions in the upper airways and throat.

Finally, try not to frown or grimace when auscultating the chest as, although it is probably due to a tight stethoscope, it may give the mother the impression that there is something wrong with the baby's heart.

Head and neck

Looking first at the outline of the head you will encounter a variety of shapes and sizes caused most often by bruising and swelling as the head is squeezed through the birth canal, but the shape returns to normal within a few days. Only babies born by Caesarean section

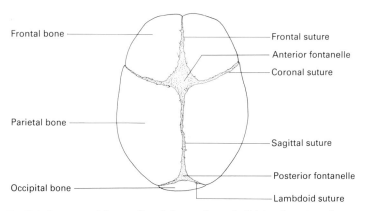

Fig. 7.2 Sutures and fontanelles of the newborn skull (view from top of head).

have perfect round heads. The head can be subject to many injuries at birth and it is important to examine for these (see p. 70).

Asymmetry may also be due to long-term moulding in the uterus if the fetus lies in an awkward position. This flattening of the occiput and opposite frontal region usually grows out within the first 2 years and is known as plagiocephaly.

Next feel for the sutures and fontanelles (Fig. 7.2). The depression felt between two skull bones consists of connective tissue and is known as a suture. When more than two bones meet the wider space forms a fontanelle. Sutures are normally less than 1 cm wide but can be proportionately larger in a larger head. The gap may disappear if the bones overlap one another due to moulding during birth. It is important to differentiate this from premature closure of the sutures (craniosynostosis) when they are heaped up and form a ridge, as this latter condition distorts the skull and may impair brain growth (Fig. 7.3).

The anterior fontanelle is variable in size but can be up to 3–4 cm long. It closes at about 18 months but there is a wide normal range. The smaller posterior one is finger-tip size (0.5–1 cm in diameter) and closes at about 3 months. Normally the anterior fontanelle is slightly concave and pulsates but it becomes tense and bulges when there is raised intracranial pressure and this can be indicative of meningitis. A marked depression can be a sign of dehydration.

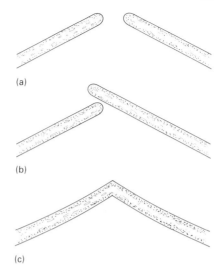

Fig. 7.3 How skull sutures may feel at birth. (a) Normal suture (gap felt between bones). (b) Moulding (bones overlap). (c) Craniosynostosis (suture closed prematurely).

Sometimes you can feel a distinct widening of the sagittal suture between the anterior and posterior fontanelles which is known as the third fontanelle. It is round or oval in outline and is situated at the junction of the middle and posterior third of the suture. Although more commonly found in Down's syndrome it also occurs in normal babies.

Look at the ears next. Small, abnormally shaped or low-set ears are often a pointer to dysmorphic syndromes. A low-set ear is defined as one in which the top of the ear is below a line drawn back from the outer corner of the eye.

The nose usually has a flat almost non-existent bridge at birth. This can give the false impression that the eyes are widely spaced apart (hypertelorism) and, if there is any doubt, measure the distance between the inner canthi which should be between 1.5 and 2.5 cm.

Babies breathe through their noses and it only takes a small quantity of mucus to impair breathing. It can also make feeding difficult as a clear nasal airway is needed for effective sucking. Very snuffly babies can be helped by gentle nose suction. Flaring of the nostrils is a sign of respiratory distress.

Look in the mouth and inspect the tongue, and run your finger along the hard palate to ensure there is no cleft.

A careful examination of the eyes is important but since the lids are usually quite puffy and swollen in the first few days this can be difficult. Never try to prise open the lids as you will not succeed and it looks rather brutal. Babies open their eyes spontaneously when they are being fed and sometimes while sucking on a finger. They also usually open them when held upright over the mother's shoulder. If you do not get a proper view you must try again later.

Inspect the sclera, iris and pupil. The newborn sclera has a bluish tinge whilst a yellow colour is a good sign of hyperbilirubinaemia in a dark-skinned baby. Caucasian babies usually have blue-grey eyes and it takes at least 6 months for the iris to take on the final colour. The darkly pigmented eyes of Afro-Caribbean and Asian babies are usually apparent at birth.

Full fundoscopy is not necessary but it is mandatory to look at the pupils through the fundoscope from a distance to see the red reflex. Look straight on at the baby's pupils from a few feet away. You should see a bright red/orange glow from the pupils which is the reflection of light from the back of the retina. This is not difficult and is a crucial screen for congenital cataracts characterized by pupils which appear dull grey rather than bright orange.

Persistent nystagmus is never normal. A baby's eyes may wander in the first day or so, but after this any remaining squint is abnormal and needs assessment by an ophthalmologist.

The neck is very short in the newborn and in reality impossible to examine.

Chest
Note any chest wall deformities such as funnel chest or pigeon chest. A prominent xiphisternum is a common and harmless finding. Feel the clavicles for any lumps which may indicate a fracture.

Check the position of the nipples and look for the presence of accessory nipples. A minor degree of breast engorgement is common and a few drops of colostrum are sometimes secreted.

If the respiratory rate has not been recorded by the nurses then it should be counted. This must be done for a full minute and is more accurately done with a stethoscope than by observing the chest movement. If repeated values are required then it is easiest to use a Graseby MR10 Respiration Monitor which counts the rate. The upper limit of normal is 60 breaths/minute. The pattern of breathing should also be noted. Subcostal or intercostal recession (i.e. indrawing of the chest wall) is a sign of respiratory distress. Chest movement should be symmetrical.

The apex beat should be palpated although this can be difficult in the newborn. In a well child it is unnecessary to count the heart rate as long as you can recognize the normal rhythm of 110–160 beats/minute from a bradycardic rate of less than 100.

Abdomen

First of all inspect the abdomen. Major defects such as gastroschisis and omphalocoeles will have been noted at birth. Sometimes there is a protrusion running down the centre of the abdominal wall which is caused by divarification of the recti muscles and is of no significance.

You should examine the abdomen gently for abnormal masses but wait until the baby is relaxed. The liver is normally palpable 1–2 cm below the right subcostal margin. It is just possible to feel the spleen in some infants and with care the kidneys are also palpable. If either are very easy to feel then they are probably enlarged. The bladder is an abdominal organ at this age and is usually only palpable if there is a distal obstruction.

The remnant of the umbilical cord should be inspected for signs of infection. It is often slightly sticky and should be cleaned and then dried with powder containing an antiseptic. The stump separates and falls off after about a week.

Anus and genitalia

Check the position of the anus. The patency will usually have been confirmed by the midwife who will have taken the rectal temperature after delivery.

Inspect the genitalia. If the scrotum is poorly developed the possibility of undescended testes should be considered. It is important to palpate both testes and look for hydrocoeles and inguinal herniae which are common (see p. 95). The penis is normally 2.5–3.5 cm long at birth whilst the foreskin is adherent to the glans penis and no attempt should be made to retract it. A hooded prepuce suggests a hypospadias which is a common abnormality (see p. 97).

In girls, the clitoris is often prominent and if the infant is premature the labia minora are also seen easily but later they are covered by the labia majora. A grey-white mucoid vaginal discharge is often seen and sometimes a small amount of vaginal bleeding due to oestrogen withdrawal is noticed after 5–7 days. Prolapse of the vaginal mucosa is a common normal finding. It results in a mucosal tag seen around the posterior vulva which soon disappears.

Ambiguous genitalia indicate that the baby requires urgent attention (see p. 111). If there is any doubt at all over the sex of a baby then the parents must wait for the result of chromosome analysis. Although this may be difficult for them, incorrect guesses can have serious consequences. The social implications are enormous and the parents must be encouraged not to name the baby until the true sex is known.

Part of the examination is to find out about the passage of stools and urine.

Stools
Simple observation of the nappy may give you all the information you need. Meconium is the sticky greenish-black material produced for up to 2 days and it is important to record whether the baby has passed any within the first 48 hours, as a delay may indicate intestinal obstruction or even Hirschprung's disease. A baby may have passed large amounts at birth in which case there is little produced in the first day or so. Sometimes a white plug is passed before the first meconium. For the next few days, 'changing stools' are produced which are softer and greenish-brown. Finally, the 'milk stools' appear. In the case of breastfed babies these resemble bright yellow seedy mustard and may be quite soft or even liquid, but they are firmer and browner in bottle-fed children.

Urine
Urine is usually passed within a few hours of birth. Rarely, and

probably due to the passage of urine at delivery, no further urine may be passed for a further 36 hours. After this time the possibility of posterior urethral valves in a boy must be considered (see p. 109). Poor feeding and dehydration is another possibility. Early urine samples often contain urate crystals which leave red streaks on the nappy and cause alarm as they are mistaken for blood. The stream produced is also important as a poor one may indicate urethral valves but a thin jet stream can also indicate a meatal stenosis.

Femoral pulses
These are difficult to feel in the newborn but you should persevere. Weak or absent femoral pulses coupled with normal pulses in the arms are indicative of a coarctation of the aorta (see p. 232). If this is suspected then the blood pressure must be measured in all four limbs which is easy and quick using an electronic doppler machine such as the Dinamap. In the first few days the pressure in the legs is normally 15–20 mmHg lower than in the arms. Greater differences indicate a narrowing of the aorta below the origin of the ductus arteriosus. A lesion above this level may produce no differences.

If the femoral pulses are normal, routine measurement of blood pressure in healthy babies is not indicated.

Limbs
Upper limbs
First look at the hands and check that there are neither too many nor too few fingers and thumbs and that they have the correct appearance. Also check that the nails look normal. Abnormalities of the hands are a common feature of many dysmorphic syndromes. Look also at the creases on the palm. A single palmar crease (simian crease) is found commonly in Down's syndrome (45% cases) but also occurs in 4% of normal children in whom it is of no significance.

Place your little finger in the baby's palm from the ulnar side, and he should grip it tightly as part of the grasp reflex.

Check the arms are held in a normal position and that there are active movements.

Lower limbs

Look at the feet in a similar way to the hands checking the toes. The feet are often held in an abnormal position due to the way they have been squashed against the wall of the uterus. This 'postural talipes' is easily differentiated from a true talipes as the postural type can always be straightened passively and usually reverts to normal in a few weeks.

If you gently stroke the side of the foot, the child should demonstrate the Babinski's sign, the toes splay out with the big toe pointing upwards (dorsiflexion). The big toe points downward once the child can walk.

Look at the spontaneous movements in the legs and their posture at rest. The tibiae often appear to bow outwards with an internal rotation but this is a normal appearance.

The back

You should now pick up the baby and turn him over which will probably wake him if he is still asleep. As you do this it provides a good chance to assess his truncal tone. Support him under his chest and abdomen with your left hand whilst your right hand steadies his back. Look at how he hangs there and you will be able to differentiate a floppy baby who lies like a rag-doll from one who lies stiffly out like a flat board and is hypertonic. This is called 'ventral suspension'; obviously minor variations from the normal are harder to detect (Fig. 7.4).

Look at the neck and along the whole back down to the natal cleft. The back of the neck is a common site for the stork bite simple naevus whilst the lower back is where you find Mongolian bluespots (see p. 98). Check there are no pits or sinuses over the sacrum or coccyx. A midline hairy naevus overlying the lower spine may indicate a spina bifida occulta or other spinal lesions and further advice is needed.

A major spina bifida will have been seen at birth but run your hand down the spine and check that the vertebrae feel normal. This usually makes the baby arch his back and you can also see if the spine has a normal free movement. Also check there are no fixed deformities such as a kyphosis or scoliosis.

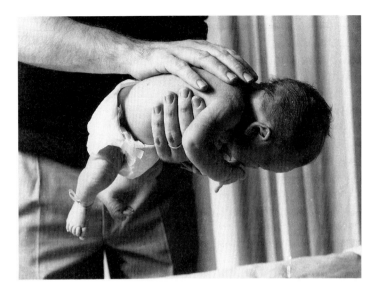

Fig. 7.4 Ventral suspension.

Hips

Detection of congenital dislocation of the hips (CDH) is one of the most important parts of the examination and is a true example of preventive screening. However it always makes the baby cry and looks rather unpleasant so explain to the mother why you are doing this. Management of CDH is discussed on p. 112.

Ideally the baby is relaxed and lying on his back. The procedure should never be performed with the baby wearing a nappy! Observation may reveal asymmetric skin creases in the groin or an abnormal leg posture which may be a clue to abnormal hips. Note also the degree of femoral abduction at rest.

With the knees and hips flexed to 90°, grip the greater trochanter with the thumb anteriorly on the inner thigh and the fingers posteriorly over the greater trochanter itself. Do not hold the knees alone as this produces dangerous leverage. Hold each leg in slight abduction then try to move each femoral head gently forwards into or backwards out of the acetabulum. After this,

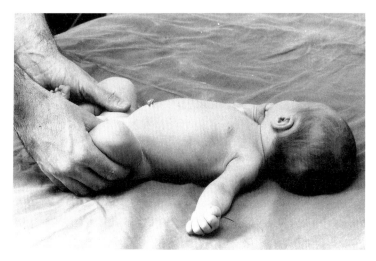

Fig. 7.5 Examining the hips.

slowly abduct each hip from the midline out to 90° and back again (Fig. 7.5).

Remember that hips dislocate in a posterior direction so results of your examination tend to fall into one of three groups:
1 No abnormal movement of femoral head — normal hip.
2 Femoral head moves forwards — dislocated hip.
3 Femoral head moves backward — dislocatable hip.
Movement of the femoral head is the only reliable sign of CDH and this may be accompanied by a distinctive 'clunking' sensation as the posteriorly dislocated hip is returned to the acetabulum (i.e. slips forwards). This finding is known as Ortolani's sign and the 'clunk' is obvious. The dislocatable hip is diagnosed when the femoral head is pushed out of its socket in which it is held in an unstable fashion (i.e. slips backwards), this is a positive Barlow's sign.

The hips can be made to abduct to 90° in the first 2 days of life with the outside of the knees almost flat on the sheet. Whilst limited abduction suggests dislocation, a normal degree of abduction does not exclude the diagnosis.

Frequently one encounters a grating sensation or a clicking

sound. This is the 'clicky hip' and is due to ligamentous movement. As long as the hip is otherwise normal this is of no significance and disappears after a few weeks. Creaks sometimes come from the knees. If in any doubt over the clinical signs, the hips should be examined by someone more experienced, and if there is still uncertainty, an ultrasound examination performed.

Unfortunately not all dysplastic hips are detected by examination and if the child is at increased risk (i.e. family history of CDH or extended breech presentation) or has other bony or neuro-muscular abnormalities, then again it is safest to arrange an ultrasound of the hips.

Head circumference

It is convenient to leave this to last since it does tend to make many babies cry, and also if you do it too early in the examination the figure is forgotten by the time you come to write the notes.

The head will have been measured at birth but this is usually inaccurate due to moulding and oedema. Now is a better time to

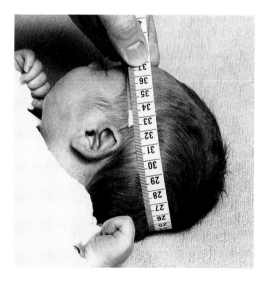

Fig. 7.6 Measuring the head circumference.

get the baseline measurement as much of the swelling will have gone down.

Use a disposable paper tape measure (one for each child) but beware as the edges are often very sharp. In theory you should measure the occipitofrontal circumference (OFC) but in practice if the head is still misshapen then take the largest circumference (Fig. 7.6). It is best to take the average of two or three measurements. The normal range is 32–38 cm.

It is reasonable to ask the mother to dress the child when you have finished. However if she has just had a Caesarean section she will still be uncomfortable and relatively immobile so you should offer to do it yourself.

It is quicker to write up the notes at the end but do so in detail as they may well be referred to at a later date.

8: Minor Congenital Abnormalities

Minor abnormalities are frequently found on routine examination. A thorough search for other abnormalities is necessary as a minor defect may be a clue to an underlying more serious problem. 13% of children have a single minor anomaly and only 3% of them have an associated major defect. However of the one in 200 children that have three or more minor anomalies, 90% have a major malformation. However minor or common, any abnormality still causes anxiety to the parents and a full explanation and reassurance is necessary.

HEAD

Asymmetric crying facies
When the baby cries, one corner of the mouth does not move downwards and outwards giving an asymmetric appearance, but at other times only minimal asymmetry is noticeable. It is due to hypoplasia or absence of the depressor anguli oris muscle. It can

be confused with a facial palsy but is only apparent on crying and the rest of the facial muscles are normal so there is no problem with forehead wrinkling or eye closure. There may be some improvement over time as other muscles compensate, and is then only noticeable when the child cries or grimaces. An association with cardiac anomalies has been reported but this may be a coincident pairing of two common disorders rather than a true link.

Accessory auricles
A small pedunculated skin tag is seen anterior to the ear. If the pedicle is extremely narrow and has no cartilage within it, the tag can be tied off at the base with a silk thread. It is painless and the tag will soon drop off. Otherwise they should be removed surgically when the child is older as this gives a better cosmetic result.

Preauricular pit
A small sinus may be seen just anterior to the auricle. It is commoner in girls and is of no significance.

Tongue tie
The frenulum runs from the floor of the mouth to the tongue. Despite popular myth it does not hinder feeding nor affect speech. It should be left alone and surgical removal will simply replace the frenulum with scar tissue.

Neonatal tooth
Occasionally one or two lower central incisors have already erupted at birth. They have only a little enamel, and no roots so are often only loosely attached. It is best to remove the tooth to avoid the risk of inhalation but this should wait until the tooth is loose. This does not affect normal dentition.

Ranula
This is a bluish cyst found in the floor of the mouth at the base of the tongue. It is a mucus retention cyst and many disappear spontaneously. The larger cysts may need surgical treatment.

Epithelial pearls (Epstein's pearls)
Tiny epidermal cysts resembling miniature pearls are commonly seen on the hard palate around the midline. They may occur in clusters at the junction of the hard and soft palate and also occur sometimes on the alveolar margin. They disappear spontaneously and should be left alone.

CHEST

Accessory nipples (polythelia)
These resemble a miniature nipple and may be found anywhere along the embryological mammary line that extends from the axilla down to the groin. Sometimes there is no more than a tiny pigmented spot. They are of no significance but occasionally accessory breast tissue also develops (polymastia), usually in the axilla. This breast tissue needs removal as it undergoes all the hormonal changes associated with the breast.

Pectus excavatum (funnel chest)
This is a fixed depression of the mid-sternal region and anterior part of the ribs. In the newborn it must be differentiated from sternal recession associated with respiratory distress. As the child grows the deformity becomes more noticeable and is often accompanied by rounded shoulders and a slight kyphosis. Respiratory symptoms are sometimes reported but are probably psychological in origin, and it can be surgically corrected for cosmetic purposes.

Pectus carinatum (pigeon chest)
The sternum is projected forwards giving a bowed chest. The deformity is harmless and cosmetic surgery is possible when the child is older.

ABDOMEN

Umbilical hernia
This hernia at the umbilicus is easily reducible and usually contains omentum and intestine. It is present in 20% of the

newborn and is even commoner in Afro-Caribbean babies (60%). 90% will spontaneously regress but repair is advisable if still present at 5 years. It must be differentiated from a paraumbilical hernia which is found in the midline above or below the umbilicus, as these do not regress and require surgery.

Umbilical granuloma

This is not a congenital lesion but is acquired. It is an overgrowth of granulation tissue found at the centre of the umbilicus once the cord has separated. It is probably due to low-grade infection and produces a sero-sanguinous discharge. Best seen by pulling back the surrounding skin of the umbilicus, it is an irregular pink lump. Treatment is by application of the tip of a silver nitrate stick to the granuloma, which may need to be repeated. Great care must be taken not to apply the silver nitrate to normal skin as this causes a superficial burn and leads to infection. The normal skin can be protected by covering it with Vaseline jelly. It needs to be differentiated from an umbilicial polyp which is a remnant of the vitello-intestinal duct. This has a smooth, rounded, shiny red appearance and requires surgical removal.

GENITALIA

Hydrocoele

This is a collection of fluid in the scrotum which cannot be emptied. It varies in size and with the larger ones the testis may not be palpable. It can be differentiated from an inguinoscrotal hernia as it transilluminates, although in practice this is difficult to see in the newborn. It does not extend above the inguinal ring. The fluid is resorbed and the smaller ones have disappeared within a month. Follow-up is not necessary as long as both testes have been felt. Parents should be reassured that the fluid does not harm the testis.

Inguinal hernia

These are more commonly found in premature babies and in boys. A loop of bowel usually enters the scrotum (inguinoscrotal hernia) but can be easily reduced. The scrotum does not transilluminate and bowel sounds may be heard within the scrotum. There is a risk of the hernia becoming irreducible and strangulating, so surgery is advisable for all cases, within a few days of diagnosis. Parents must be told to consult a doctor immediately at the first signs of strangulation or obstruction (red painful mass in the groin, vomiting or abdominal distension). Any girl with bilateral inguinal herniae should have chromosomal analysis before surgery as 2–4% will have testicular feminization syndrome. In this syndrome, the external genitalia are female, but the hernia contains a testis.

Undescended testes
An undescended or ectopic testis is present in 3% of fullterm babies. It is even more common in premature babies in whom it usually descends within the first three months of life. The testis is usually palpable high in the scrotum or in the superficial inguinal pouch. Sometimes it can be gently 'milked' out of the inguinal canal. If the testis is impalpable it may be either in the inguinal canal, intra-abdominal or absent. 25% of cases are bilateral and if neither testis is palpable (cryptorchism), the question of intersex arises. An ultrasound examination can be useful for locating the testes. The cremasteric reflex is poorly developed at birth so it is unlikely that the testis is retractile. Patients with an undescended testis (in contrast to an ectopic one) have a small underdeveloped scrotum on the affected side. An inguinal hernia frequently accompanies an undescended testis. Patients need follow-up and many of the testes will have descended within the first year. If not, orchidopexy is necessary, and although the timing varies, most surgeons will operate by 2 years of age.

Neonatal torsion and infarction
This presents as an enlarged scrotum with a bluish discoloration. Sometimes a hard mass is felt and it is rarely tender. It is noticed soon after birth but is not due to birth trauma. It almost invariably occurs prenatally and although the aetiology is unclear, it is probably a primary vascular event. Sometimes the testis infarcts spontaneously without torsion. Urgent surgical exploration is required and although the testis is necrotic by this stage, the other side can at least be fixed in place and its survival ensured.

Hypospadias

This is a common abnormality with an incidence of one in 160. There is a hooded prepuce and the urethral meatus is usually found at the base of the glans penis. The meatus may however be situated anywhere along the ventral surface of the penis down as far as the perineum. If there is a good stream of urine and no curvature of the penis (chordee) then immediate treatment is not required. The patient should be referred to a plastic surgeon and it should be stressed to the parents that circumcision must not be performed in the meanwhile. Surgery is not always necessary but if it is, then it is usually carried out at age 2–3 years.

SACRUM

Sacral pits

A sinus is commonly found in the midline overlying the coccyx in the natal cleft. By pulling at the skin on either side it is nearly always possible to see whether the pit is blind ending. However even if the end can not be seen, as long as the sinus is overlying the coccyx or is below it, it is harmless as it does not communicate with the spinal canal. A midline pit anywhere else along the spine may have a fistulous connection to the dural space and needs investigation and excision as it can lead to meningitis.

HANDS AND FEET

Syndactyly

Syndactyly is an incomplete separation of two or more digits. Severity varies from fusion of the complete digit to a minor degree of webbing. In the hand it most commonly affects the middle and ring fingers and minor syndactyly of the second and third toes is considered a normal variant. Surgical separation and skin grafting is performed when the child is 4 or 5 years old.

Extra digits (polydactyly)

This condition, which is often familial, ranges in severity. There may be a fully formed extra digit complete with a nail which needs surgical excision. Alternatively the digit may be no more than a skin tag, usually on the lateral aspect of the hand or foot.

If the tag has a thin base and contains no bone or cartilage, it can be tied off with a silk thread, otherwise it should be excised by a plastic surgeon for cosmetic reasons.

Clinodactyly
This is a curved finger due to hypoplasia of the middle phalanx. It usually affects the little finger which curves inwards. Whilst sometimes familial and benign, it is found more commonly in Down's syndrome.

Toe deformities
These are very common and often familial. As well as syndactyly and clinodactyly, the toes may be of asymmetric length, there may be overlapping of toes, hammer toes or a wide gap between the big toe and second toe. Many deformities are of no significance but shoe fitting may become a problem and advice can be sought when the child is older. The toenails may also be hypoplastic but this is considered a variant of normal.

Postural talipes
See Chapter 9, p. 113.

SKIN

Mongolian blue spots
These are patchy accumulations of pigment over the buttocks and lower back, and are occasionally seen on the limbs. They are a normal finding in non-Caucasian babies, particularly those of Asian and Afro-Caribbean origin but also occur in other babies (e.g. Greek, Italian). They become less obvious as the rest of the skin darkens once the child gets older. Their only significance is that they can be mistaken for bruising.

Café-au-lait patches
These are non-raised pale brown patches with distinct edges. They are of no significance and are what is commonly thought of as a 'birthmark'. However, if there are more than five patches greater than 0.5 cm then a diagnosis of neurofibromatosis must be excluded (after puberty they must be over 1.5 cm).

Simple naevus
Diffuse capillary naevi are pink macular areas (non-raised) that do not blanch but tend to redden when the baby cries. They are very common and are seen on the forehead, upper eyelids and the back of the neck. They are also known as salmon patches and the mark on the neck is the 'stork bite'. Although the lesions on the face fade over the first year, a naevus on the neck tends to persist.

Depigmented patches
These small areas of pale skin are uncommon in the newborn. They are of no significance although rarely patches on the trunk or limbs may be associated with tuberose sclerosis (epilepsy, adenoma sebaceum rash, mental retardation).

Strawberry mark
This is a capillary haemangioma that is not usually present at birth. It starts as a small red spot within the first month and grows rapidly over several weeks. It becomes a bright red raised lump with small white speckles hence its name. Strawberry marks are commonly found on the head, neck and trunk but can occur anywhere on the body, and are commoner in premature babies. They grow over the first year then almost all of them undergo complete or partial spontaneous resolution. This starts at 6–12 months, and is complete in 50% by 5 years and 70% by 7 years. 80% disappear completely. The haemangiomas are asymptomatic and only require treatment if they are close to vital structures such as on the eyelids where they may obstruct eye opening. In these cases, a short course of systemic steroids may speed up resolution. Occasionally they can bleed or ulcerate if subjected to trauma.

Cavernous haemangioma
This is similar in nature to a strawberry mark but involves deeper layers of dermis. Most commonly, the lesion is a mixed strawberry and cavernous haemangioma. It comprises large vascular elements with venous anastamoses. It is a bluish-red raised lesion with indistinct edges. Cavernous hemangiomas do not grow as rapidly, and although they resolve spontaneously they do not

usually disappear completely. When very large, they may cause thrombocytopenia due to sequestration of platelets.

Port-wine stain
This is a flat capillary haemangioma which ranges in colour from pink to purple. Port-wine stains can occur anywhere but tend to be on the face and may be quite extensive. They are present at birth and grow with the child. Unfortunately they do not resolve although they may fade slightly. Results of cosmetic treatment are usually unsatisfactory but disguise with make-up can be considered when the child is older.

When the naevus occurs in the distribution of the trigeminal nerve and does not cross the midline, there is a possibility of an associated intracranial vascular anomaly (Sturge–Weber syndrome) which may lead to epilepsy or hemiplegia. There is also an association with congenital glaucoma when the port-wine stain is on the face. The glaucoma is usually asymptomatic at first but the eye may appear large with clouding of the cornea.

Hairy naevus
This is a pigmented area covered by dark fine hair. They occur only rarely in the newborn but require immediate referral to a plastic surgeon for removal. If treated in the first week of life, while the pigmented cells are still superficial, debridement is all that is required and this leaves no scar. The very rare giant hairy naevus has a considerably increased risk of malignant change before puberty.

FURTHER READING

Spitz L, Steiner GM & Zachary RB (1989) *A Colour Atlas of Paediatric Surgical Diagnosis.* Wolfe Medical Publications Ltd, London.
Verbov J (1988) *Essential Paediatric Dermatology.* Clinical Press Ltd, Bristol.

9: Major Congenital Abnormalities

Congenital abnormalities account for almost 25% of childhood deaths. Most serious abnormalities are immediately recognizable and this chapter stresses those conditions in which early intervention is necessary. Abnormalities are often multiple so if one defect is found you must look carefully for others.

CENTRAL NERVOUS SYSTEM

Neural tube defects

These are the commonest major congenital abnormalities in the UK. The overall incidence is 2–3 per 1000 births but there are wide geographical differences. They are more common in South Wales and Northern Ireland than in South-East England or East Anglia. The incidence is decreasing due to antenatal screening, very often leading to termination of pregnancy. The risk of having a second affected child is increased tenfold but folic acid supplements before conception may reduce this risk.

Myelomeningocoele

A myelomeningocoele is a neural tube defect in which there is an abnormal development of the spinal cord associated with deficiency of the dorsal laminae and dorsal spines of the vertebrae (spina bifida). This leaves a flat or raised plaque of exposed neural tissue in the midline over the spine. Although most commonly found in the lumbosacral region, it also occurs in the thoracic spine. There is a major risk of meningitis and trauma to the delicate nervous tissue so it must be covered with a sterile dressing. Suitability for surgery depends on the overall prognosis and the baby needs urgent assessment in conjunction with a paediatric surgical centre. If there are no active movements of the legs and the anus is patulous it is very likely that the infant will be incontinent of faeces and urine and unable to walk unaided. The high thoracolumbar lesions and defects larger than four vertebrae are indicators of a worse prognosis. Other such indicators are the presence of kyphoscoliosis, hydrocephalus or other

101

associated anomalies. Frequently there are accompanying bony abnormalities such as congenital dislocation of the hips or clubfoot. Renal anomalies are also often present.

Meningocoele

These lesions are similar to myelomeningocoeles except that they are always covered by the meninges and often by skin as well so that the neural tissue is relatively protected. There is a better prognosis than with a myelomeningocoele as neurological problems of the lower limbs and hydrocephalus are unusual. However, minor bladder dysfunction is not uncommon.

Spina bifida occulta

This bony abnormality, which is due to failure of fusion of the dorsal spines, causes no neurological problems. It is very common and usually noted as a chance finding on X-ray. Occasionally there is an overlying hairy patch or naevus and this may be associated with tethering of the spinal cord or an intraspinal lesion such as a dermoid or lipoma. It is these associated conditions which can lead to a mild spastic gait or bladder problems as the child grows.

Cranium bifidum defects

An encephalocoele is a rare cranial lesion which usually occurs in the occipital region. Large defects are untreatable as it results in the loss of too much brain tissue.

If the defect contains no neural tissue (meningocoele) then the prognosis is good once skin cover is obtained. However if the lesion is large, hydrocephalus may occur after surgery.

Anencephaly

There is absence of the cranial vault and most of the brain. The baby is either stillborn or dies shortly after birth.

Hydrocephalus

Hydrocephalus is present in over 80% of infants with a myelomeningocoele. Other congenital causes include malformations (e.g. aqueduct stenosis) and infections (e.g. toxoplasmosis). Acquired causes include intracranial haemorrhage and neonatal meningitis. The diagnosis may be obvious from the appearance of a large head with wide sutures, dilated scalp veins and 'setting-sun' eyes. The occipitofrontal head circumference should be serially measured, preferably by the same person. Plotting the values on a growth chart will show the head to be above the 97th centile and growing away from the centile lines. Ultrasound through the anterior fontanelle will monitor the degree of ventricular dilatation and a CT scan may reveal the aetiology. Progressive hydrocephalus needs to be treated in order to reduce the intracranial pressure. A catheter with a one-way valve is inserted into the cerebral ventricle and drains into the superior vena cava or into the peritoneal cavity.

Microcephaly
This is a small head which is particularly noticeable since the forehead is so small in relation to the baby's face. The head circumference is usually well below the third centile. There is an invariable association with mental impairment. Aetiology is usually unknown but it may be related to congenital infections such as rubella or cytomegalovirus. Genetic counselling is essential as there is an increased risk in some families.

CLEFT LIP AND CLEFT PALATE

These abnormalities are frequently associated and the incidence of cleft lip with or without cleft palate is between one in 700 and one in 1000 live births. The chance of having a second affected child is increased 40-fold. A cleft lip may be unilateral or bilateral and is due to failure of the maxillary process growing towards the midline to fuse with the premaxilla. The rare central cleft lip is associated with midline abnormalities of the brain.

Minor degrees of cleft palate can be easily missed if the hard palate is not inspected and palpated. A bifid uvula is a clue to the presence of a submucosal cleft in which there is a muscular defect covered by mucosa which leads to impaired mobility of the soft palate. Symptoms are identical to those of a complete cleft, namely regurgitation of feeds through the nose and difficulty with speech.

Most of the infants can feed normally from the breast or bottle. If there are difficulties, then special teats and spoons should be tried. The lip is usually repaired at 3 months and the palate at 1 year. The condition is often very disturbing for the parents and bonding may be a problem. It is helpful to show them photographs of other children before and after their operations. Cosmetic results are usually good, but many of these children are prone to recurrent otitis media and they all need follow-up to monitor speech and hearing.

Pierre Robin syndrome
This syndrome is relatively common and is due to hypoplasia of the mandibular area. There is a small jaw (micrognathia), a wide posterior cleft palate and a tendency for the tongue to fall backwards and occlude the airway (glossoptosis). Feeding difficulties are also common. The baby must be nursed in a prone position and may required a nasal airway. As the infant grows the risk of respiratory obstruction decreases and the palate is repaired at 3 months.

CONGENITAL CATARACTS

The lens opacification is either present at birth or appears soon afterwards. Cataracts may be inherited in an autosomal dominant manner. They are also associated with congenital infections (e.g. rubella) and metabolic disorders (e.g. galactosaemia or hypocalcaemia). A completely opacified lens is easy to detect as it appears dullish grey and the eye loses the red reflex (see p. 84). Smaller opacities however are not easy to detect. Surgery is necessary before 3 months otherwise sight will never develop in that eye. Long-wearing contact lenses are fitted to the baby soon after operation.

CHOANAL ATRESIA

In this rare condition, the nasal passage is blocked either by bone or a membrane. If unilateral, it may go undetected for years and the child presents with persistent nasal discharge and sinusitis or a blocked nose. However when bilateral, it presents in the newborn with respiratory distress, particularly during feeding. Diagnosis is confirmed by an inability to pass a nasogastric tube down either nostril. An oral airway may be necessary in an emergency and the baby needs urgent referral for surgery.

CONGENITAL HEART DISEASE

See Chapter 20.

ALIMENTARY TRACT

Oesophageal atresia and tracheo-oesophageal fistula
The incidence of oesophageal atresia (OA) is one in 3000 live births. In 7% of cases there is no accompanying tracheo-oesophageal fistula (TOF) but the commonest abnormality is an OA with a fistula from the trachea to the distal part of the oesophagus (85%). The fistula may connect instead to the upper oesophageal pouch, both the upper and lower oesophagus or finally, there may be a fistula connected to a normal oesophagus, known as an H-type fistula (Fig. 9.1). Almost half the babies have associated anomalies, usually cardiac, anorectal, skeletal or renal.

The diagnosis must be excluded whenever there is maternal hydramnios which may be caused by an inability of the fetus to swallow. Otherwise the baby usually presents with excessive mucus and frothing at the mouth. If the baby is fed there may be respiratory distress with choking or a cyanotic episode. Diagnosis is confirmed by gently passing a radio-opaque feeding tube (size FG 10) down the oesophagus. It will be impeded at approximately 10 cm from the lips but if the tube is too soft, it can coil up in the oesophageal pouch giving a false impression that it has passed into the stomach. With the tube in place, a plain X-ray of the chest and abdomen is taken — use of contrast media is unnecessary and dangerous. The tip of the tube will be situated at the level of the second to fourth thoracic vertebrae and the presence of gas in the bowel confirms a fistulous connection.

The baby needs immediate referral to a neonatal surgical centre. In the meanwhile he should not be fed but should be

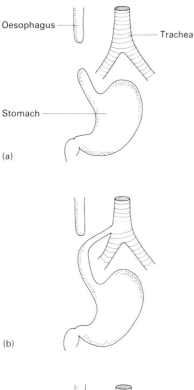

Oesophagus

Trachea

Stomach

(a)

(b)

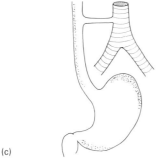

(c)

Fig. 9.1 Types of oesophageal atresia and tracheo-oesophageal fistula (rarer types not shown). (a) Oesophageal atresia without fistula (9%). (b) Fistula to lower pouch (85%). (c) H-type fistula. No oesophageal atresia (4%).

started on maintenance IV fluids. Pass a double-lumen Replogle tube into the oesophageal pouch and keep it on continual suction to avoid secretions spilling over into the lungs. If this is not available, use a large nasogastric tube and aspirate it every 10 minutes. Send 10 ml of the mother's blood with the baby for cross-matching as well as a consent form for operation. Repair can sometimes be done at a single operation unless the gap between the upper and lower portions of the oesophagus is too great, in which case it is a two-stage procedure.

Intestinal obstruction

There are many congenital causes of intestinal obstruction which are dealt with in Chapter 13. These include:
• duodenal atresia, stenosis and webs;
• jejunal atresia and stenosis;
• malrotation;
• volvulus;
• meconium ileus and plugs;
• Hirschsprung's disease.

Anorectal anomalies

Imperforate anus occurs in one in 2500 births. The anus may be situated in an ectopic position and is not patent. Diagnosis is obvious from simple inspection. In the more serious form, the bowel terminates above the level of the levator ani muscles. This 'high' lesion is often accompanied by fistulae from the bowel to the urethra or vagina and meconium may be passed from these sites. In the less serious 'low' form, the anus may simply be covered by skin. Differentiation can be made with a lateral X-ray of the abdomen once air has reached the lower bowel (at least 12 hours of age). The baby is kept with his bottom raised for a few minutes before the X-ray is taken and a radio-opaque marker is placed on the skin over the site of the anal dimple. The level of the gas shadow is then related to bony landmarks and the skin marker. The baby requires a nasogastric tube, IV fluids, and surgical referral. With the high lesion, a colostomy is necessary and often several operations are required before the repair is satisfactory. Repair of the low lesion is relatively simple.

Another anomaly sometimes seen is a rectal prolapse. Usually only 2–3 cm of mucosa prolapses, it appears on straining and reduces spontaneously. The importance is that it occurs in 10% of children with cystic fibrosis and may be the presenting feature. Alternatively the full thickness of the rectum may prolapse, and this type usually accompanies neuromuscular disorders such as spina bifida.

RENAL

Hydronephrosis

The kidney is easily palpable but examination alone will not reveal the cause of the enlargement. Hydronephrosis is due to obstruction of the urinary tract anywhere along its length. Most commonly the obstruction is at the pelviureteric junction and it is bilateral in 20% of cases. An ultrasound examination should be performed and this is urgent if the condition is bilateral. Outcome depends on the degree of obstruction. The infants are prone to urinary tract infections and gross bilateral obstruction may need to be relieved surgically.

A degree of pelvicalyceal dilatation is commonly detected antenatally on ultrasound but usually resolves spontaneously before birth (see p. 34). If however some dilatation persists then the baby must have a follow-up ultrasound before discharge from hospital, and another one 6 weeks later (the first one may miss a degree of dilatation if the baby only passes small volumes of urine in the first 48 hours).

Cystic kidneys

Enlarged palpable kidneys may be due to cystic disease. Renal disease is often associated with hypertension so it is important to monitor the blood pressure in any child with renal anomalies.

Multicystic and dysplastic kidneys
The dysplastic kidney is formed by primitive renal tissue and cysts. A multicystic kidney consists of many different sized cysts and presents as a lobulated mass in the loin. Both abnormalities result in a non-functional kidney so if the condition is bilateral it is lethal. When unilateral, urinary infections are common and there are often other abnormalities in the urinary tract.

Infantile polycystic kidneys
This is an autosomal recessive condition in which both kidneys

are enlarged and cystic. It usually presents as bilateral loin masses. There may be accompanying cystic disease of the liver and pancreas, and if the lungs are also involved there are respiratory problems at birth. Renal failure ensues and it is lethal unless transplant is possible.

Adult polycystic kidneys
This is an autosomal dominant condition so there should be a family history. The cysts are slow growing so the condition does not normally present until early adulthood, but sometimes enlarged kidneys are palpable in the newborn.

Posterior urethral valves

This is the commonest form of lower urinary tract obstruction in boys. The presenting feature may be a poor urinary stream or failure to pass urine in the first 36 hours; however a good stream does not exclude the diagnosis. There may be abdominal distension due to an enlarged bladder and the kidneys may be palpable due to hydronephrosis. The baby may also present with a urinary tract infection or, rarely, urinary ascites following a leak from the urinary tract. Severe renal damage may be present at birth due to back pressure during intrauterine life. Diagnosis is confirmed by a micturating cystourethrogram and ultrasound of the renal tract. Bilateral nephrostomy followed later by removal of the valves is required.

Potter's syndrome

This lethal syndrome has an incidence of one in 4000 births. It is characterized by bilateral renal agenesis or other severe abnormalities of the kidneys which leads to oligohydramnios. This results in pulmonary hypoplasia and the baby is either stillborn or dies within a few hours. There is a raised respiratory rate with subcostal recession similar to respiratory distress syndrome. The babies have a low birthweight with limb contractures and the recognizable Potter's facies in which there is a compressed appearance with a furrowed forehead and large, floppy, low-set ears.

ABDOMINAL WALL

Exomphalos

An exomphalos (omphalocoele) is a hernia into the base of the umbilical cord. In exomphalos minor the defect is less than 5 cm in diameter and herniated intestine is seen through a transparent amniotic membrane. This contrasts with a true umbilical hernia which is covered by skin. In an exomphalos major, the defect is greater than 5 cm and the sac contains intestine as well as liver. There is a high incidence of associated major abnormalities (e.g. cardiac, gastrointestinal, renal) which accounts for the overall mortality of 25–30%. Exomphalos is also associated with chromosomal abnormalities (e.g. Trisomy 13, Trisomy 18) and the Beckwith–Wiedemann syndrome (macroglossia, gigantism, hypoglycaemia, polycythaemia).

The defect should be wrapped in clingfilm and covered in a sterile dressing. A nasogastric tube is left on free drainage and IV fluids commenced. Surgical closure is necessary but a large defect may require a staged procedure. An alternative treatment is to paint the sac with an antiseptic solution such as mercurochrome. This results in formation of an eschar and subsequent epithelialization over a number of weeks. The resulting umbilical hernia is then repaired after 18 months.

Gastroschisis

In this defect the intestines protrude through the abdominal wall to the right of the umbilicus. There is no covering sac and the bowel has a dull oedematous appearance. The immediate problems are heat and fluid loss from the bowel. The baby should be intubated immediately and paralysed with pancuronium to avoid overdistension of the bowel. The intestines should be wrapped in clingfilm and covered with swabs that are soaked in warm sterile saline (these must be changed when they cool down). The bowel must be supported but should be handled gently. A Replogle tube is left on continuous suction or a nasogastric tube on free drainage. IV fluids are commenced and 10–20 ml/kg albumin given to combat fluid loss into the bowel. The baby is then ready for immediate transfer to a surgical centre. Primary closure may be possible otherwise the bowel is suspended in a sac and reduced into the abdominal cavity over 1–2 weeks prior to skin closure.

Exstrophy of the bladder

There is failure of development of the anterior wall of the bladder and the lower abdominal wall. This leaves the posterior wall of the bladder and ureteric openings exposed and the bladder mucosa is continuous with the skin. There is a complete epispadias — in boys the urethra is an open strip of mucosa on the dorsum of the penis while in girls, the urethra appears as a broad transverse slit with the clitoris split in two. There is also wide separation of the symphysis pubis and the upper renal tract may also be abnormal. Referral to a paediatric urologist is essential.

AMBIGUOUS GENITALIA

There are many rare causes of ambiguous genitalia. These include:
• genetic (e.g. true hermaphrodites, mosaics);
• hormonal (e.g. maternal androgen or progesterone ingestion, testicular feminization syndrome; testosterone deficiency);
• endocrine (e.g. congenital adrenal hyperplasia);
• structural (e.g. severe perineoscrotal hypospadias, dysmorphic syndromes).
It is most important to determine whether the baby has testes or ovaries and ultrasound examination may be helpful. Blood should be sent urgently for chromosomal analysis. Never guess at the sex of the baby.

Congenital adrenal hyperplasia

Congenital adrenal hyperplasia (CAH) (adrenogenital syndrome) refers to a group of autosomal recessive disorders in which one of the enzymes responsible for cortisol and aldosterone synthesis is missing. The overall incidence is one in 5000 and over 90% cases involve lack of 21 α-hydroxylase. Affected females are obviously virilized so this diagnosis must be considered at birth. All virilized girls must have daily checks on plasma and urine electrolytes until a diagnosis is made. However males may not present until they succumb to an adrenal salt-losing crisis in the second week. Diagnosis of CAH is made by finding raised levels of 17-hydroxyprogesterone and ACTH in the blood but it may take up to 2 weeks to get the results.

Treatment is with hydrocortisone (15–25 mg/m^2/day orally). Salt losers also require: fludrocortisone (0.25 mg/m^2/day orally); sodium chloride (2–4 g/day orally).

Monitor these factors daily: weight, blood pressure, plasma and urinary electrolytes.

A salt-losing crisis is an emergency and presents with vomiting, hypotension and weight loss. It is associated with hyponatraemia, hyperkalaemia and often hypoglycaemia. Immediate treatment is:
• IV 0.9% saline at 150 ml/kg/day;
• IV glucose as necessary;
• IV hydrocortisone 50 mg;
• oral fludrocortisone 25–50 μg.

In almost 10% of cases of CAH the enzyme missing is 11 β-hydroxylase which presents with virilization and hypertension.

SKELETAL

Congenital dislocation of the hips

The incidence of dislocated and dislocatable hips in the first 2 days of life is one in 100 live births. Without universal screening the incidence of established congenital dislocation of the hips (CDH) is one in 1000. It is four times commoner in girls and rare in premature babies. There is often a family history and there is a degree of racial predisposition, being commoner in Northern Italy and the Balkans. Other risk factors are breech presentation, oligohydramnios, myelomeningocoele and the presence of other bony or neuromuscular abnormalities. CDH is due to under-development of the acetabulum and head of the femur.

Joint care with an orthopaedic surgeon is essential. Dislocated hips are reduced then splinted in a flexed and abducted position on the second day for 6–12 weeks. The splint, which consists of a malleable metal frame covered in waterproof padding, must be kept on continuously. The position must be adjusted regularly to take into account the child's growth that alters the normal degree of abduction, otherwise there is a risk of avascular necrosis of the femoral head. If the hips are irreducible surgical reduction may be necessary. Hips that are dislocatable may be splinted immediately or can be left for 3–6 weeks as many of these will resolve spontaneously.

Despite screening, dislocated hips are still missed. The child does not present for several months and if the abnormality is bilateral, it may not be apparent until he starts to walk. Late treatment is difficult, it involves long-term splinting and often several operations. A perfect result is often not obtained and this leads to early osteoarthritis.

Talipes (clubfoot)
Postural talipes is common and is due to the foot being pressed up against the wall of the uterus. The foot has a full passive range of movement and the mother is taught to manipulate the foot after each feed. It will usually revert to normal after a few weeks.

In contrast, the foot with structural talipes has a limited range of movement. The ankle is held in an equinus position, while the hindfoot is inverted and the forefoot adducted (talipes equinovarus), so that the sole of the foot is turned inwards. Dorsiflexion of the foot is reduced. The incidence is one in 800 births, it is commoner in males and it is bilateral in half the cases. The foot should be strapped, within 24 hours of birth, into the straightest position that can be obtained without undue force and the baby needs an orthopaedic referral. Management consists of serial strapping and splints and in the more severe cases serial plaster casts and even corrective surgery may be necessary.

CONGENITAL INFECTIONS

Some microorganisms can have a devastating effect on the fetus while causing only minor illness in the pregnant mother. The defects produced tend to depend on the developmental stage which the fetus has reached when infected. The commonest congenital infections with proven teratogenic effects are CMV, rubella and toxoplasmosis. Severely infected babies present with low birthweight, jaundice, hepatosplenomegaly and thrombocytopenic purpura. In addition some of the infections produce malformations more particular to them and these are listed below. Diagnosis is confirmed by finding specific IgM in the baby's blood. Since this antibody is too large to cross the placenta it can only have been produced by an infected fetus. Other congenital infections are dealt with in Chapter 2.

Cytomegalovirus

Although affected babies are usually asymptomatic at birth, some can be acutely ill with pneumonitis and convulsions as well as the features described above. Other abnormalities include chorioretinitis, microcephaly, and cerebral calcification (on X-ray). Late features include hepatitis leading to liver cirrhosis and progressive neurological deterioration leading to mental retardation, deafness and cerebral palsy. Congenital CMV is the commonest infective cause of mental retardation. CMV can be isolated from a fresh specimen of urine, and although up to 3% of newborn excrete the virus only a minority are affected. The anti-CMV drug ganciclovir can be considered for acute severe illness but has not yet been fully evaluated in neonates.

Rubella

Common features include congenital cataracts, congenital heart disease (especially patent ductus arteriosus), nerve deafness and mental retardation. In addition there may be punctate retinopathy, myocarditis, osteitis (X-ray changes at the metaphyses of long bones), and rarely glaucoma. Some children may be affected by deafness alone. There is no specific treatment and the infants may shed the virus for many months. In order to prevent this condition, rubella vaccine is now given to all children aged 12–18 months as part of the MMR (measles/mumps/rubella) immunization schedule.

Toxoplasmosis

This is caused by the protozoa *Toxoplasma gondii* which is associated with cats and undercooked red meat. It primarily damages the central nervous system with chorioretinitis leading to blindness, convulsions, hydrocephalus and cerebral calcification. Therapy with spiramycin, pyrimethamine and sulphadiazine is possible but has unpleasant side-effects.

CHROMOSOMAL ABNORMALITIES

Down's syndrome

Down's syndrome has an overall incidence of one in 660 births, and is the commonest malformation syndrome. The incidence increases with maternal age; it is one in 1500 for mothers under 30 years and one in 100 for those aged 40–44. However most affected babies are born to younger women as fewer older women have babies. 94% of cases are due to Trisomy 21, the remainder being translocations or Trisomy 21 mosaics. The overall risk of recurrence is 1% but is higher if one parent is a translocation carrier (see p. 14).

The most striking features are the facial appearance and hypotonia and although diagnosis is often obvious, it must be confirmed by chromosomal analysis. The principal features are:
• hypotonia with protruding tongue and hypermobile joints;
• flat facial profile with flat occiput (brachycephaly), palpebral fissures with Mongoloid slant (upwards and outwards), prominent epicanthic folds, white speckling of the iris (Brushfield's spots), small abnormal ears, third fontanelle;
• excess skin on the back of the neck, dry skin;
• single palmar crease, short incurved little finger, distal palmar triradius;
• wide gap between the first and second toes with a plantar crease between them.

The presence of one of these features does not necessarily mean a baby has Down's syndrome, rather it is the clustering together of several characteristics that suggests the diagnosis. For example, prominent epicanthic folds, Brushfield's spots, a third fontanelle and a single palmar crease may all occur in normal babies.

Congenital heart disease is common (40%) particularly atrioventricular canal defects or a ventricular septal defect. There is also an association with duodenal atresia and Hirschsprung's disease. The children have short stature. They have a variable degree of mental retardation (IQ usually 25–75, mean 50) but many are now integrated into normal schools.

Trisomy 18 (Edward's syndrome)
The incidence of this lethal syndrome is one in 2000 births. The few survivors are mentally retarded. Babies are small-for-dates and often premature or postmature. Other features are a narrow small head, short palpebral fissure, low-set malformed ears, small jaw and a high-arched palate. There are also flexion deformities of the fingers and prominent heels. Congenital heart disease, renal anomalies and cleft lip and palate may also occur.

Turner's syndrome
These girls have a missing X-chromosome (XO) and the incidence is one in 5000 births. The principal features are ovarian dysgenesis and short stature. In the newborn the best diagnostic sign is non-pitting oedema of the feet and hands. Other features are webbing of the neck or loose skin folds at the back of the neck, low hairline, broad chest with widely-spaced nipples, congenital heart disease (particularly coarctation of the aorta) and renal anomalies.

OTHER SYNDROMES

Congenital hypothyroidism
The incidence of congenital hypothyroidism is one in 3500 births. Most cases will be diagnosed from the screening programme that measures TSH (thyroid-stimulating hormone) or thyroxine in the blood spots on the Guthrie card (see Appendix 6). Most of the neonates have a small or absent thyroid gland. If there is a goitre it may be due to one of the rare inherited enzyme defects or maternal ingestion of anti-thyroid drugs or iodide. The clinical signs are sluggishness, poor cry, slow feeding, dry skin, low temperature, large fontanelles due to delayed osseous maturation and persistent jaundice. Diagnosis is confirmed by a high plasma TSH level. Treatment is with 1-thyroxine 10 µg/kg/day.

Fetal alcohol syndrome

This is a difficult syndrome to recognize in the newborn but a maternal history of high alcohol intake should alert the paediatrician. The babies are usually growth retarded with a small head. Other features are short palpebral fissures, maxillary hypoplasia, a smooth philtrum with a thin smooth upper lip, a small nail on the little finger and hirsutism. The babies are often irritable and the children become hyperactive, clumsy and may have a reduced IQ.

BREAKING THE NEWS

It is a terrible shock for parents when their new baby is born with an abnormality, especially when life-threatening or disfiguring. The way the situation is handled by the medical and nursing staff at the beginning has a great impact on how the parents cope. The parents should be seen together, so if an abnormality is found, some indication must be given to the mother so that arrangements can be made to see both parents. If the problem is likely to be a long-term one, it is particularly important that a senior member of the paediatric staff who is likely to continue the long-term care should speak to the parents from the start. If a junior member of the staff has had limited experience of a particular problem, it is better to tell the parents that he needs to seek further advice rather than guess at the answer. Parents often cling to the first opinion and may find it more difficult to accept the more experienced views later. It is possible to give a statement of the facts, for example that there is an abnormality of the spine, with the assurance that a more senior member of the staff will come soon to discuss the problem in more detail.

A member of the nursing staff should always be present, as he or she is likely to be asked all the questions again as soon as the doctor has left. Ideally the interview should take place in a quiet room without telephone or bleeps, and adequate time must be set aside. The diagnosis, which may only be presumptive at the time, should be explained in terms the parents can understand. Remote possibilities need not be discussed, for example if the

probable diagnosis is a ventricular septal defect, it is not necessary to explain the outside chance of there being multiple cardiac
abnormalities. In discussing management, the help and support
that will be given by social workers or physiotherapists should be
stressed from the beginning. The parents should be advised to tell
their relations and friends the diagnosis rather than hide it. In
considering prognosis, the positive aspects should be stressed
with as much optimism as possible. Unnecessarily pessimistic
prognosis based on out-of-date information can alter a mother's
attitude to her baby. On the other hand do not give false hope.

Many parent-run support groups exist for specific conditions,
and the address as well as any leaflets prepared either by these
groups or the hospital should be given to the parents. It is often
easier for them to read the information in their own time prior to
seeing the doctor again. Several meetings are necessary as it is
hard for distressed parents to take in too much information at
once. If at all possible, the baby should be kept alongside the
mother in the maternity ward as separation from her baby will
only worsen the situation.

A meeting with a clinical geneticist should be arranged for the
parents. Recurrence risks can often be given precisely and with
many conditions prenatal screening can now be offered.

FURTHER READING

Duckworth T (1984) Congenital malformations — congenital dislocation of the
    hip. In: *Lecture Notes on Orthopaedics and Fractures*, 2nd edn, pp. 150–8.
    Blackwell Scientific Publications, Oxford.
Jones KL (1988) *Smith's Recognizable Patterns of Human Malformation*. WB
    Saunders Co., Eastbourne, Philadelphia.
Sadler D (1990) *Langman's Medical Embryology*. Williams & Wilkins, Balti-
    more.
Spitz L, Steiner GM & Zachary RB (1989) *A Colour Atlas of Paediatric Surgical
    Diagnosis*. Wolfe Medical Publications Ltd, London.

10: Small Babies

Babies are considered to be small or low birthweight (LBW) when they weigh less than 2.5 kg (5.5 lb). Very low birthweight (VLBW) babies weigh less than 1.5 kg. In the UK, 6–7% of babies are LBW.

The baby may be small because he is born too soon. When the gestational period is less than 37 completed weeks he is considered preterm or premature. About 5% of pregnancies are spontaneous preterm deliveries, with 2% being born before 32 weeks.

On the other hand, he may have reached fullterm but be small because he has not grown properly. A baby who is growth-retarded is 'small-for-dates' (SFD), i.e. has a birthweight less than that expected for the gestational age. There are growth charts which give the centiles of weight, length and head circumference for different gestational ages (see Appendix 1). The definition of SFD is not unanimous, with many people defining it as a birthweight less than the tenth centile. It is probably better to consider those babies less than the third centile to be small for dates, as fewer normal babies will be included in this definition. Some premature babies are also small-for-dates.

DIAGNOSIS

The length of gestation is calculated from the first day of the mother's last menstrual period. This may, however, be unreliable if the mother has irregular periods. Gestational age may have been confirmed at the routine 18-week ultrasound by measuring the biparietal diameter of the head of the fetus. Later ultrasound examinations are unreliable for assessing gestational age. Diagnosis during pregnancy of intrauterine growth retardation (IUGR) has been discussed on p. 33.

Once the baby is born, there are scoring systems that utilize both neurological development and certain external features of the baby to estimate the gestational age. With experience, estimates can be obtained that are reliable to within 1 week. The system developed by Dubowitz and Dubowitz is outlined in Appendix 4. The assessment should not be carried out until the baby is at least 6 hours old and need only take 10 minutes to perform. The presence or absence of neonatal reflexes may also be a guide (see Appendix 3).

Clinical differentiation between preterm and SFD babies may be difficult but there are certain pointers. Preterm babies have thin, red, shiny skin, which is often covered in soft hair (lanugo), especially on the back and shoulders. Because of poor muscle tone, they are very floppy and lie with a frog-like posture. The ears have little cartilage and are very soft. The genitalia are poorly developed, boys have a small scrotum with undescended testes, whilst girls have very prominent labia minora and an enlarged clitoris.

The appearance of small-for-dates babies depends to a certain extent on the cause. Assuming the baby is undernourished but otherwise normal, they tend to be long and thin. They have dry, lax skin, and the nails are often long. Muscle tone is usually normal and although they look small, they behave in a way appropriate to their gestational age.

CAUSES

Preterm babies

Most spontaneous preterm births are not associated with any identifiable cause. In some cases there is a known aetiology and the following are some examples:
• cervical incompetence which also often leads to spontaneous abortion in the mid-trimester;
• an abnormal fetus, particularly when accompanied by polyhydramnios;
• multiple pregnancy which commonly ends prematurely. The median gestation for twins is 37 weeks and for triplets is 33 weeks;
• polyhydramnios (see p. 28);
• abnormal membranes which are prone to rupture due to their reduced tensile strength;
• maternal infections, particularly chorioamnionitis associated

with group B β-haemolytic streptococci;
• antepartum haemorrhage.

There are also certain maternal factors which are associated with premature delivery. These are young or old age, low socioeconomic class, smoking, short stature and being under psychosocial stress. If the mother has already had a premature baby, the risk of her having another one is tripled.

The premature labour may sometimes have been induced by the obstetrician for the sake of the mother or the baby. For example, if the mother is in danger from severe pre-eclampsia or the baby is severely affected by IUGR or rhesus incompatibility.

Small-for-dates babies

There are many factors associated with growth-retarded babies:

1 Genetic background is important as small parents usually have small babies. The standard fetal and neonatal growth charts may be inappropriate for certain families and racial groups.

2 Placental insufficiency may be idiopathic but is often the end result of other adverse factors, particularly maternal hypertension.

3 Maternal hypertension particularly if associated with proteinuria. The hypertension may have been pre-existing or due to pre-eclampsia.

4 Other maternal illnesses, such as renal disease, sickle cell disease, cyanotic heart disease.

5 Major congenital abnormalities and chromosome abnormalities often result in small babies, examples include Trisomy 21, osteochondrodysplasias, Potter's syndrome and anencephaly.

6 Congenital infections such as rubella, cytomegalovirus and toxoplasma.

7 Drugs given for maternal illness such as carbamazepine, phenytoin and sodium valproate may be responsible but it is not always possible to separate the effect of the drug from the effect of the illness itself. Narcotic drug addiction also results in poor growth but the lifestyle of a drug addict may be the overriding factor.

8 Excessive alcohol intake even if it does not lead to fetal alcohol syndrome.

9 Smoking during pregnancy retards growth in the third trimester.
10 Maternal diet has little effect unless the mother is suffering from chronic malnutrition.

COMPLICATIONS

Many of the problems and hence the management of small babies are similar, whether they are preterm or growth-retarded. However certain complications are more likely to occur in one group than the other.

Preterm

Hyaline membrane disease is due to surfactant deficiency and causes respiratory distress (see p. 207). If it is mild, the baby may only need to be given oxygen in a headbox, but often ventilatory support is needed.

Intracranial haemorrhage commonly occurs in preterm babies and is a major cause of death and neurological handicap when severe. The haemorrhage may be intraventricular, intracerebral (into the brain substance itself), or subarachnoid. Unless severe, the haemorrhage is not usually accompanied by symptoms and only detectable by a cranial ultrasound examination directed through the anterior fontanelle. The baby may, however, present with a sudden collapse, becoming pale, hypotensive and apnoeic. This may be followed by a fall in haemoglobin level. Other symptoms are irritability (or sometimes undue lethargy), poor or increased muscle tone and convulsions (see p. 239).

Infection in a small baby may be very insidious and should be suspected if there are any symptoms, however slight. If the nursing staff have the slightest anxiety about any infant, even in the absence of abnormal signs, full investigation is warranted (see p. 183). Preterm babies are particularly susceptible because of their immature immune system, thin skin that is easily damaged and their repeated exposure to invasive procedures (such as intravenous and intra-arterial cannulae, central lines, endotracheal tubes).

Cross-infection can be a problem unless scrupulous handwashing is carried out by all medical staff before and after touching each infant. Ideally any baby who develops an infection should be barrier nursed in a separate cubicle. Babies transferred from another hospital should be isolated until skin swabs are reported to be negative, particularly for MRSA (methicillin-resistant *Staphylococcus aureus*). Staff with an infection such as a cold, a boil or a coldsore should not be at work on a neonatal unit.

Jaundice is very common in preterm babies, who are also more susceptible to the long-term effects on the basal ganglia (kernicterus). Phototherapy is required at lower serum bilirubin levels than in fullterm babies (see p. 173).

Hypothermia (see p. 124).

Fluid and electrolyte imbalance is a problem as the thin skin leads to a marked evaporative fluid loss particularly if the baby is under a radiant heater. This in turn can lead to a marked hypernatraemia. Alternately the immature kidney fails to conserve sodium resulting in hyponatraemia. Electrolyte balance needs daily monitoring, and in a sick infant this may need to be done even more often.

Feeding difficulties are common as babies under 34 weeks gestation do not suck properly. In addition, they have a poor cough reflex so care must be taken to avoid aspiration into the lungs. When the baby is unable to feed by mouth, frequent small-volume feeds are given down a nasogastric tube. Alternatively, a continuous feed administered by a pump can be given nasogastrically. This avoids overdistending the stomach which can cause an apnoeic episode or a fall in arterial oxygen saturation. Sometimes a nasojejunal tube is used if the infant has a problem with gastro-oesophageal reflux or vomiting. Either the mother's expressed breastmilk or low birthweight formula milk is used.

Extra vitamins are required once milk is started (e.g. Abidec 0.6 ml daily); this contains vitamins A, B, C and D. After the second week, oral iron should also be given, for 6 months.

If the infant is very sick, enteral feeding should be avoided. In the short term, IV fluids (10% glucose with added sodium and potassium) are given (see p. 145). However, after a few days, extra calories are required and then total parenteral nutrition (TPN) should be given. Glucose amino acid solutions with lipid are used which also contain vitamins and the essential minerals. TPN is best administered via a central line but scrupulous aseptic techniques handling the solutions are essential due to the risk of septicaemia.

Small-for-dates babies

Hypoglycaemia is a particular problem in undernourished babies due to lack of glycogen stores. This can be prevented by early feeding with milk which should be continuous or every 3 hours for the first day. Asymptomatic hypoglycaemia must be detected by performing a BM stix test every 3 hours for the first 24 hours. If the baby is feeding well and the BM stix are consistently above 2 mmol/l then the testing can stop after 24 hours. If any of the readings have been lower then monitoring should continue and be reviewed after another 24 hours. For further management see p. 162.

Hypothermia can start very quickly in small infants. Heat loss may be considerable because they have a large surface area in relation to body weight. Also they are deficient in subcutaneous fat which acts as insulation. In addition, preterm babies lack the 'brown fat' that is present in the fullterm baby and which can be rapidly metabolized to produce heat. The thin skin of a preterm baby also allows rapid heat loss.

Hypothermia is associated with a raised metabolic rate and an increased energy and oxygen requirement. A cold baby is prone to acidosis, hypoxia and hypoglycaemia. Respiratory distress is worsened due to the deleterious effect of cold on surfactant function. There is a marked increase in mortality associated with hypothermia.

Prevention of hypothermia starts in the delivery room. Firstly the room must be kept warm, even if it is uncomfortable for the midwife and mother. The baby is dried quickly, wrapped in warm blankets and a hat should be put on him. The overhead radiant heater should also be turned on in case prolonged resuscitation is required. The baby should be taken to the neonatal unit without delay in a portable transport incubator that is kept prewarmed. If the baby is to be transferred to another hospital, extra care must be taken to avoid hypothermia. Babies who are going to the postnatal ward should have their temperature checked 3-hourly for the first 24–48 hours.

If the baby is sick, he can be nursed on an open incubator under a radiant heater, as this allows ease of access. There will be increased water loss through the skin and extra fluid must be given (30 ml/kg/day). Clingfilm placed above the baby's body may help prevent excess water loss.

Normally the child will be put into a closed incubator which will provide a high constant environmental temperature. The incubator temperature is initially set at 35°C. It is then adjusted according to the baby's rectal temperature which should be maintained between 36.8–37°C. Many incubators are servo-controlled and will adjust themselves according to the reading from a probe placed on the baby's skin. However with the larger babies, the baby becomes cold before the heater comes on and this can potentially cause cold stress. Babies are nursed naked at first and a perspex heat shield may be put over them to further reduce heat loss.

Once an incubator temperature of 31°C (or 30°C for preterm babies) is all that is needed to maintain a normal rectal temperature, the baby may be put into a cot. This would only be considered if the weight is over 1.6–1.8 kg and the baby is otherwise well. If the birthweight is over 1.8 kg in a growth-retarded baby who is not premature, he should be able to maintain his body temperature in a cot on the postnatal ward.

Polycythaemia with a venous PCV (packed cell volume) over 65% is sometimes seen in SFD babies. Management is discussed on p. 176.

Hypocalcaemia with a serum calcium <1.75 mmol/l may occur in SFD babies. It is usually asymptomatic but they may be jittery or even have convulsions (see p. 240). Treatment with oral calcium supplements is sufficient if the child is asymptomatic (5–10 ml/day of 10% calcium gluconate divided into the feeds).

WHERE SHOULD SMALL BABIES BE NURSED?

If at all possible, the baby should be kept with his mother to avoid the effects of maternal separation (see p. 40). To a large extent this depends on the facilities in the hospital.

If the local unit can not cope with very premature babies (usually less than 32 weeks), the baby should be sent to a tertiary referral neonatal unit. This is either done before delivery if there is time (*in utero* transfer), or after birth (*ex utero* transfer). *In utero* transfers are probably the safest for the baby as long as there is no risk of a delivery in the ambulance. An *ex utero* transfer should only proceed once the baby is stabilized. Most special care baby units can look after babies who are over 32 weeks gestation unless the baby becomes particularly unwell.

Some hospitals also have a transitional care unit. Here the baby is kept beside the mother with greater supervision from the nursing staff. Babies over 35 weeks are suitable for transitional care, and babies over 37 weeks should be on a normal postnatal ward.

Growth-retarded babies with a birthweight <1.8 kg should be on a special care baby unit. If transitional care is available, it is suitable for babies weighing 1.8–2.5 kg. Babies over 2.5 kg can be on the postnatal ward. We would allow Asian babies with a birthweight >2.2 kg to go to the postnatal ward as this is an equivalent in birthweight centiles to 2.5 kg for Caucasian babies.

There is no target weight babies must reach before they are allowed home, although it would be most unusual under 1.8 kg. They can usually be discharged after 2–3 days as long as they are feeding well and maintaining their body temperature at a normal room temperature of 21–24°C. Prior to discharge, there is a need for a report from the health visitor about the adequacy of the home, especially the heating in the winter. It is reassuring if they are also gaining weight but it must be remembered that there is a physiological weight loss over the first three days. It is important to warn the community midwife and general practitioner before discharging small infants.

OUTCOME

The mortality rate starts to rise considerably at a birthweight less than 1.0 kg, and similarly for a gestational age under 28 weeks. Under 24 weeks the baby is not viable, but by 28 weeks there is an 80% survival rate. This rises to 95% by 30 weeks. Clearly the results are changing all the time, with advances in knowledge, equipment and drugs. Unfortunately the price is survival of more babies with severe handicap. The commonest sequelae are neurological (cerebral palsy, hearing and sight impairment), and respiratory (chronic lung disease due to bronchopulmonary dysplasia). The incidence of sudden infant death is much higher in babies born at less than 36 weeks gestation.

Growth-retarded babies have a good outcome as long as they are otherwise normal and have an uncomplicated delivery. Unfortunately they are prone to birth asphyxia and there is a slightly increased risk of major handicap such as cerebral palsy. Up to a third have minor neurological problems which may be due to impaired brain growth in the last trimester. Many of these babies who are uniformly small continue to have a subnormal growth rate and never catch up with their peers. Administering growth hormone does increase the growth rate but the effect on final height is not yet known.

FURTHER READING

Chamberlain G (1992) *ABC of Antenatal Care.* British Medical Association, London.
Roberton NRC (1986) *A Manual of Neonatal Intensive Care.* Edward Arnold, London.

11: Twins

TYPES

There are two types of twins. Firstly, a single egg that has been fertilized by a single sperm (to form the zygote) divides in two and each part undergoes complete embryogenesis. This results in monozygotic (MZ) uniovular identical twins. The splitting of the zygote may occur at different stages. At the earliest stage, it results in separate implantation in the uterus so each twin has its own placenta and chorionic sac. More commonly, the splitting occurs at a time that leads to a common placenta and chorionic cavity but separate amniotic cavities. Rarely (in 4% cases), the split occurs at a late state, and the babies share a single placenta and a common chorionic and amniotic cavity.

Should the separation occur at a very late stage or be incomplete, the result is conjoined (Siamese) twins. This is fortunately extremely rare but survival after surgery is sometimes possible.

The commonest type of twins arise when two eggs are simultaneously shed and both are fertilized by separate sperm. These twins are known as dizygotic (DZ) or binovular. They have different genetic constitutions and are non-identical, although may, of course, be the same sex. The two zygotes implant separately and each has its own placenta, amnion and chorionic sac. Occasionally, the placentae are so close that they fuse together, and the chorionic sacs may do likewise.

Parents always want to know whether the twins are identical soon after delivery. It may be be possible to tell them by examining the placenta and membranes. If there is a single chorionic sac then they are definitely monozygous. However, if there are separate chorionic sacs, they may be either MZ (when the split occured very early) or DZ. In this case, differentiation will not be possible at this stage if they are of the same sex, although sometimes they clearly look different.

FREQUENCY

Approximately 70% of twins are DZ, whilst 30% are MZ. In the

UK, the prevalence of twin births is one in 105 deliveries. The frequency of MZ twins is fairly uniform, but DZ twins vary markedly between races, being 50 times commoner in Nigeria than Japan. DZ twins are also commoner in women over 35 years of age, and there may be a family history of twins. There has been a sharp increase in multiple pregnancies over the last 10 years. This is due to fertility drugs that stimulate the ovary to shed more than one egg at a time and also due to the ever increasing use of *in vitro* fertilization. There is also an increasing number of older women having babies.

EFFECT ON THE MOTHER

The majority of twin pregnancies are diagnosed at the 18-week routine ultrasound examination. This means that it is now rare for the mother to have a sudden surprise at delivery. Nevertheless it is still an extra burden to have two babies to look after and there may be financial difficulties.

The mother has worse symptoms of pregnancy such as nausea and vomiting, backache and leg swelling. There is also an increased incidence of hypertension, anaemia and antepartum haemorrhage, with consequent effects on the fetus.

EFFECT ON THE BABIES

Perinatal mortality rate
This is increased fourfold compared to singletons and is higher in MZ than DZ twins. The main causes are prematurity, intrauterine growth retardation, congenital abnormalities and complications at delivery.

Prematurity
Twins are 4–5 times more likely to be born prematurely and the median gestational age is 37 weeks. The cause is thought to be due to the extra stretching on the uterine wall and there is little that can be done to prevent the onset of premature labour. The risks to the babies of prematurity have been discussed in the previous chapter.

Intrauterine growth retardation
The average birthweight of a twin is less than that of a singleton at fullterm. The fall-off in growth tends to occur in the last trimester. It is not always easy to detect and serial ultrasound examinations are necessary. Disparity in size of the two babies may be due to twin-to-twin transfusion (see below). Management of a growth-retarded twin is the same as for a singleton, however the babies should be kept together. If one needs to be on a neonatal unit they should both be there, or alternatively, more leeway should be given to allow the smaller twin to remain on the postnatal ward with the larger baby.

Congenital abnormalities
The risk of a major congenital abnormality is double that for singletons. It is 2–3 times commoner in MZ twins than DZ and when they share the same amniotic cavity, malformations are common. In particular, there is an increased incidence of neural tube defects, congenital heart defects and chromosomal abnormalities such as Turner's and Klinefelter's syndromes. With all twins, a detailed anomaly ultrasound scan should be performed at 20 weeks and a fetal cardiac scan at 21–24 weeks. Amniocentesis may also be required but the rate of miscarriage following this procedure is 3% which is six times higher than with singleton pregnancies.

Complications at delivery
When the twins are delivered vaginally, the mortality rate for the second twin is higher than the first. Malpresentations are common and there is a greater risk of cord prolapse. Labours are often prolonged. A paediatrician should always be present at the delivery, and if they are premature there should be one paediatrician for each baby.

Twin-to-twin transfusion
When MZ twins share the same placenta, they may also have vascular interconnections. In almost 20% of MZ twins this results in an unbalanced circulation so that one twin bleeds into the other one. The recipient baby is polycythaemic and may appear plethoric. The donor twin is anaemic and in severe cases may be

hydropic and even die *in utero*. The recipient twin is usually bigger than the other twin. At birth, if there is an obvious discrepancy in size or one twin seems paler, the full blood count should be checked. Initially a PCV can be done on a sample of capillary blood.

If the anaemic twin has a Hb <12 g/dl he should be transfused with packed cells. A Hb of 12–14 g/dl should be aimed for and the volume of transfusion is calculated as follows:

$$\text{Volume packed cells (ml)} =$$
$$\text{Weight of baby (kg)} \times 3 \times \text{desired rise in Hb (g/dl)}.$$

If the child is asymptomatic, fully cross-matched blood should be used, and is given over 3–4 hours. If, however, the anaemia is very severe and the baby is hypotensive, an initial transfusion of 15–20 ml/kg of uncross-matched O-negative blood should be given over 10 minutes.

Polycythaemia is diagnosed by spinning the blood sample for at least 10 minutes in a capillary tube and reading the PCV which is the same as the haematocrit. Polycythaemia is defined as a venous PCV >65%, or, a capillary blood sample PCV (from a heel-prick) >70%. For the complications and management, see p. 176.

Feeding

The mother will spend much of the time feeding her two babies. If they are bottle-fed, this is not a particular problem. However breastfeeding needs careful planning and once the babies' weights are over 3–4 kg, milk production may be insufficient to exclusively breastfeed them. At first, they can feed simultaneously from each breast but they should alternate sides in case one breast is producing more milk. Later, they can either alternate a breastfeed with a bottlefeed, or have a complementary feed of formula milk after each breastfeed.

TRIPLETS OR MORE

Previously, triplets arose from a combination of MZ and DZ twinning. Two eggs were fertilized simultaneously, and then one underwent a split so that three babies were produced. At present, the commonest cause is *in vitro* fertilization with implanting of multiple eggs. The use of drugs such as clomiphene given for ovulatory failure has also resulted in an increased in multiple pregnancies. The natural incidence of triplets is one in 10 000 pregnancies and quadruplets is one in 500 000.

The complications of higher order births are similar to twins but occur more frequently. The perinatal mortality rate is over 15% for triplets and 20–25% for quadruplets. The median gestation for triplets is 33 weeks, and IUGR is common. The arrival of three or more premature babies simultaneously places a great burden on neonatal units. It is also a tremendous amount of work for parents once the babies go home and extra help is necessary. This may be provided by grandparents and other family, friends and home helps.

12: Feeding

Feeding a newborn baby can be an extremely rewarding experience for parents. However if any difficulties are encountered it is a cause of great anxiety and many parents become concerned about the baby's weight gain. It is normal for babies to lose weight (about 5% of birthweight) over the first few days as their energy expenditure and fluid loss exceeds their intake. However birthweight should be regained within 7–10 days. A weight loss greater than 10% of the birthweight in the first 3 days may indicate a problem with the baby and should be investigated. Fortunately it is usually only a simple problem with feeding technique which is easily remedied. Once the birthweight is regained, the baby should gain approximately 30 g/day (1 oz/day) for the first 3 months. Daily fluctuations are normal so it is better to consider weight gain over a week which should average 180–210 g (6–7 oz).

BREASTFEEDING

It is current policy to encourage all mothers (with few exceptions) to breastfeed and the Department of Health launched the

National Breastfeeding Initiative in 1990. Promotion and education is best done while girls are still at school, but should be reinforced during the antenatal period. Most mothers will have made up their minds by the time the baby is born. Although mothers should still be encouraged on the postnatal ward, it is wrong to pressure them and make them feel guilty if they have decided to bottle feed.

Statistics for England and Wales show that in 1985 the incidence of breastfeeding was 65% (this is defined as the number of babies who had at least one breastfeed) which was slightly less than in 1980. However over a third had stopped breastfeeding by 6 weeks of age.

Advantages

1 The fat and protein of human milk are more easily and completely absorbed than cow's milk. Breast milk is a perfectly balanced diet for the newborn infant which can not be completely mimicked. The breast milk composition changes during the feed, the fore milk contains more water and protein whilst the hind milk contains more fat.

2 Human milk — and particularly that produced in the first few days (colostrum) — contains immunoglobulins (mainly secretory IgA) and other substances which may protect the infant against infection. These include the bacteriocidal enzyme lysozyme, lactoferrin which is an iron-binding protein that inhibits the growth of *Escherichia coli*, and interferon which has antiviral properties. Gastroenteritis is rare among breastfed babies and there are fewer respiratory infections. It does not however affect superficial skin, eye or mouth infections nor does it abolish nappy rashes.

3 Exclusive breastfeeding for the first 6 months is considered to lessen the risk of hypersensitivity to cow's milk protein although this is a rare condition anyway. Contrary to previous evidence, there seems to be no benefit conferred by breastfeeding in preventing the development of eczema or atopic asthma.

4 Mother–infant attachment is enhanced by the closeness of breastfeeding. However this assumes it is easy for the mother, and in those cases where she finds it uncomfortable or unpleasant it can have negative effects. In addition bottle feeding can also be rewarding for parents, and helps the father feel more involved with the care of his baby.

5 Breastfeeding is certainly cheap and convenient. There is no need to carry around all the paraphernalia involved in sterilizing bottles. The only problem is that only the mother can do the feeding and this is not always practical. One way round this is for her to express breast milk which can be stored frozen. Someone else can then help out without having to resort to artificial milk.

6 Although it is not necessarily causally related, the incidence of cot deaths is lower in breastfed babies.

Breastfeeding in practice
Ideally the baby is put to the breast immediately after delivery. Suckling will even help delivery of the placenta. If this is not possible, breastfeeding should start within 4 hours. The first feeds are important because if successful breastfeeding is established at this stage, it is less likely that difficulties will be encountered later. Some infants are reluctant to take the nipple initially and the mother requires strong reassurance that this occurs commonly.

It is best to feed the baby 'on demand'. The baby rooms in with the mother, with the cot placed next to her bed. She is able to pick up her baby and feed him when he cries and the mother should be encouraged to do this. At first, most babies will feed every 2–4 hours and this may increase to 10–12 feeds for 24 hours by the third or fourth day. As the baby begins to regain his birthweight and the milk becomes fuller with an increased fat content, the baby will settle down to feeding every 3–4 hours. The baby will continue to wake for feeds during the night for 6–10 weeks and this is the most tiring period for the mother. After this, he will tend to have five feeds during the day at 4-hourly intervals. It is said that breastfed babies cannot be overfed, and although some get quite fat, they tend to lose the weight later.

Although the colostrum produced in the first few days would appear rather 'thin', it provides the correct amounts of water and nutrients for the baby. It is also the part of the breast milk that has most of the anti-infective properties. The fuller milk should appear by the fourth day. The amount of milk produced varies markedly at first, but the more the baby suckles the breast, the more the milk is generated. Once feeding is fully established, the average mother produces 700–800 ml per day.

Normally a hungry baby has a strong rooting reflex, whereby when the cheek touches the mother's breast, he can find the nipple. When the corner of the mouth is touched, the head and tongue turn towards the stimulus and the lip lowers on the same side.

It is most important that the baby latches on to the nipple correctly otherwise it is most uncomfortable, even painful for the mother. The nipples can be damaged and successful breastfeeding will never be established. Although for some mothers and babies latching on to the nipple occurs totally naturally, for others help must be given. It is the sensation of the nipple against the palate that stimulates the baby to suck. In order for the nipple to reach the palate, the baby's chin must be pushed into the breast with the head tilting back and up (i.e. extending the neck). If the baby's head is overflexed, the nipple comes into contact with the lower jaw and tongue and the nose is squashed up against the breast which impedes breathing. To achieve the correct position, it is best to support the baby's back under the shoulders with the baby facing the mother. Holding the back of the baby's head will tend to make the neck flex and hinder feeding.

The baby obtains most of the milk within 5 minutes during the first week or two, and so the mother should not feel discouraged if he falls asleep at the breast after 5 or 10 minutes. Each baby will take a different time to feed but advice is needed if it exceeds 45 minutes. Babies alternate long sucks during which they swallow milk with lighter sucks that serve to stimulate milk flow through the nipple.

Complementary feeds

The practice of giving the occasional extra bottle feed to a breastfed baby should be discouraged. It is rarely necessary and should be done only in exceptional circumstances, for example when there is a truly inadequate milk supply, or a small-for-dates or asymptomatic hypoglycaemic baby who will not take to the breast. Despite the fact that complementary feeds are associated with failure of breastfeeding, half the babies are still given an extra bottle in the first week. It is usually given because the baby is thought to be hungry and the mother becomes anxious over her milk supply. However it has adverse effects since if the baby is no longer hungry, he will suckle less at the breast and then milk production is reduced further. Giving extra feeds will also undermine the mother's confidence in her ability to support the baby. In addition, the feel of a bottle teat is rather different from a nipple and when the baby is accustomed to one it may be difficult to persuade him to take from the other. Finally, one or two artificial feeds may break down the barrier to infection and possibly sensitize the gut to cow's milk protein. Extra water can be given if the infant is thirsty during the first few days.

Difficulties with breastfeeding

The commonest reasons for stopping breastfeeding are insufficient milk supply, sore nipples and a baby who does not suck properly.

Inadequate milk production. Sometimes there is insufficient milk produced and the baby is always hungry. Feeding will go on a long time and the baby will not settle and cries incessantly. Underfeeding also leads to the frequent passage of small amounts of green mucus. If the feeding technique is checked and seen to be correct it is likely that the milk supply is inadequate. Frequent breastfeeding for 24–48 hours may help increase the production but if the baby is still unsettled and has shown no weight gain then complementary feeding with formula milk is necessary. After an initial 10 minutes at the breast, the baby should be given as much bottle milk as he wants to take.

Breast engorgement can occur with excessive milk production towards the end of the first week but is unusual with demand-fed babies. The breasts look obviously engorged and are tender. It is relieved once the baby has fed and then expressing milk with an electric pump will give further relief. However if too much milk is taken off it will only encourage further production.

Cracked nipples are usually due to incorrect positioning of the baby's head so that he does not latch on to the nipple properly. Pulling the infant off the breast abruptly is another cause. The nipple becomes bruised and blistered and is extremely painful. The nipple must be rested and the milk should be expressed from that side while carrying on normal breastfeeding from the other side. Bland ointment should be applied to the nipple.

Sometimes a fissure appears at a later stage which is colonized with *Candida* infection passed on from the baby's mouth. Miconazole gel should be applied to the nipple and also to the baby's mouth.

Acute mastitis usually occurs when there has been previous damage to the nipple. There is fever, pain, flushing and induration of one breast. There is usually also axillary lymphadenopathy which helps differentiate it from simple breast engorgement. The mother should be treated with anti-staphylococcal antibiotics (flucloxacillin or erythromycin) for a week. Breastfeeding should continue, and the baby should start with the affected side in order to empty that breast. Swabs should also be taken from the baby's mouth in case he is a staphylococcal carrier.

Inadequate or inappropriate treatment can lead to a breast abscess which is indicated by the presence of a fluctuant area under the induration. Surgery will be necessary and lactation should be suppressed with bromocriptine.

Problems with the baby are usually only minor. Sometimes the baby develops intestinal hurry on the fourth or fifth day when there is plenty of milk and he is feeding often. This results in frequent loose green stools but is usually transient and no treatment is necessary. Usually the stools of a breastfed baby have a soft, bright yellow, seedy appearance. Once the baby is a few weeks old, he may only pass stools once a week which can be quite normal.

Another problem sometimes encountered is gulping. During the first feed of the day, the milk may spurt quite quickly from the breast. The hungry baby may swallow excessive air as he gulps at the fast milk flow. This can lead to discomfort with excessive crying and regurgitation. The solution is to manually express the first 30 ml of milk which can be given to the baby later.

All babies will swallow a certain amount of air with the feed which commonly causes wind, although this is less common with breastfeeding. After feeding, the baby should be sat upright with his chin supported and have his back patted gently. Another way of winding the baby is to lie him on his front at an angle with his head higher than his feet. This can be achieved by placing a pillow under the mattress. The angle encourages the air bubble to travel upwards and out. An alternative method is to support the baby by putting your hand under his stomach so that the weight of his body puts gentle pressure on the stomach which releases the wind. When a belch is finally produced, it is probably more of a relief to the parents than the baby. Parents must be encouraged not to be overzealous in their attempts to produce this belch.

Some babies will simply not suck properly at the breast. If they are seen to latch on in the correct way, and are otherwise perfectly well, there is nothing more that can be done and a bottle should be tried.

Contraindications to breastfeeding

There are few contraindications to breastfeeding. Some women have a revulsion to the idea and it would be a mistake to try and persuade them. Some of the problems with the nipple discussed above are temporary contraindications to feeding from the affected side, but feeding should normally discontinue if there is an abscess.

In the UK it is currently recommended that women who are HIV-positive do not breastfeed, as there is a small risk of transmitting the virus in the milk to a baby who may not have already been infected. This advice does not apply to developing countries where failing to breastfeed carries a much greater risk of serious infections in a baby who may already be immunocompromised.

No drugs should be taken by a lactating mother unless there are strong clinical indications. However most drugs that are essential for the mother are excreted in the milk in insignificant amounts, so breastfeeding should not be stopped unless there are specific reasons. Important drugs that should be avoided during breastfeeding are listed in the *British National Formulary*.

BOTTLE-FEEDING

Contents

The contents of formula feeds are now much closer to human milk than they were previously. The sodium and protein contents are now quite similar so that unlike the older cow's milk preparations, they are less likely to be associated with hypernatraemia, hypocalcaemia and obesity.

Formula milks have a higher content of all vitamins than breast milk, in particular vitamins D and K. They also contain extra iron as well as all the required minerals.

Most formula milks are classified into either whey dominant or casein dominant, depending on which is the dominant protein. The whey dominant types are closest to mature breast milk and tend to be used for younger babies, whereas casein types tend to be used for infants older than 4 months. The latter are often marketed as being more suitable for the 'hungry' baby and said to be more satisfying, but there is no evidence to show that one type is more suitable for babies of a certain age or appetite.

Table 12.1 gives examples of some of the commonest types of milks used in the UK. Formula milks have also been produced that are suitable for premature babies. These contain more protein and calories and have a higher sodium content.

Table 12.1 Some of the commonest types of milks used in the UK.

Manufacturer	Whey-dominant	Casein-dominant
Wyeth	SMA Gold cap	SMA White cap
Cow & Gate	Premium	Plus
Milupa	Aptamil	Milumil
Farley's	Ostermilk	Ostermilk 2

Practical advice

Despite the apparent advantages of breastfeeding, it must be said that the vast majority of bottle-fed babies thrive and come to no harm. Many mothers simply prefer to use artificial milks and they should not be made to feel stigmatized on the postnatal ward. Parents should be shown how to correctly make up the feeds and how to bottle-feed their babies. Many of the problems encountered are related to poor hygiene, inadequate sterilizing techniques and mistakes over the amount of powder used.

Making up feeds

Most hospitals use ready-made formula milk but these are not easily available for use at home and are also more expensive. Most parents will have to make up feeds from powder. The instructions must be followed carefully. The powder should be measured accurately, avoiding packed or heaped spoons. A little bit extra does the baby harm rather than any good. The ratio is always 1 scoop to 30 ml (1 oz) of water. The water must be boiled first and then allowed to cool down. Feeds can be made up for the whole day and can be kept in a refrigerator for up to 24 hours. Before feeding, the milk should be at room temperature or warmed slightly. It is dangerous to warm the bottle in a microwave oven as whilst it may feel warm on the outside, it may contain milk in the centre of the bottle that is extremely hot.

How much feed?

Bottle feeding can also be given on demand but the volumes must be measured out. A normal term infant receives 30 ml of milk per kg bodyweight during the first day. The amount is increased by 20 ml/kg each day until a maximum of 150 ml/kg is reached on the seventh day. If for any reason the baby needs more fluid (for example if he is under phototheraphy), water can be given to make up extra volume. Premature babies may receive up to 200 ml/kg/day. These figures are not rigid but more of a guideline as babies have varied appetites.

The following is an example of a typical regime for a 4-kg baby who is settled on full feeds. Volumes are given in ounces as well as millilitres as this is what most parents use:

• daily requirement: 150 ml/kg = 600 ml/day (which is the same as 5 oz/kg or 2.5 oz/lb hence 20 oz/day);

• if the baby is fed 3-hourly, he requires eight feeds per day in which case he is fed 75 ml (2.5 oz) per feed;

• if he is fed 4-hourly then he requires six feeds of 100 ml (3.3 oz); Most bottles hold 300 ml whilst the ready-made bottles of milk contain 100 ml.

The majority of feeding problems arise from overfeeding or underfeeding, so it is always important to calculate exactly what the baby is receiving.

Giving the feed

The baby should be cradled in the left arm with his head supported. The bottle is held at an angle to ensure the teat is always full of milk otherwise he will suck in too much air. He should be allowed to suck at his own speed but the feed should usually take 15–20 minutes to complete. The baby will soon develop eye contact with the person feeding him.

Sterilizing the equipment

Bottles should be sterilized in dilute hypochlorite solution (Milton). Most sterilizing solutions are made from tablets that are dissolved in tap water. The bottles should be washed, then kept in the tank of sterilizing solution until ready for use. They must then be rinsed thoroughly in boiled water before being filled with milk. Teats should be sterilized by rubbing them in a small container of salt kept for this purpose. They must be rinsed very carefully, making sure there is no salt left on them and can also be kept in the sterilizing tank. There are also electric sterilizing units available which clean the equipment with steam.

Problems

As long as sterilization of the bottles and preparation of the milk is carried out scrupulously, few problems should arise that are specific to formula milks.

If the hole in the teat is too small, the baby may have to suck hard to get any milk. As well as becoming tired too soon, he will swallow excessive air and regurgitate it later along with the milk;

this is often accompanied by bouts of screaming. It is useful to look at the speed the drops come out the teat. When the bottle is tipped up, the drops should follow each other quickly but not in a continuous stream. The hole can be enlarged with a hot needle.

The hole in the teat may be too large, in which case the baby again swallows too much air as he gulps to avoid choking. A new teat must be used.

Some babies regurgitate excessively; many of these probably have gastro-oesophageal reflux which is discussed along with other causes of vomiting in Chapter 13. Unfortunately, parents are often told to switch milks from one brand to another and many babies have been through the whole range. The formula milks are all very similar and changing brands is rarely helpful.

The infant who is given an excessive volume of milk vomits, then appears hungry so is fed even more, then cries and vomits again. To stop this cycle, the correct requirement must be calculated and if it is adhered to properly, the baby soon settles down.

If a baby refuses feeds, whether breast or bottle, it may indicate an underlying illness. Although non-specific, it can be an important symptom of serious infection such as pneumonia or meningitis, or congenital heart disease. It may of course be something minor such as a blocked nose from a cold, or thrush in the mouth which can be sore. The child must be examined carefully.

VITAMIN SUPPLEMENTS

There is still not total agreement over recommendations. Normal breastfed babies and babies fed on modern formula milks do not need vitamin supplementation. Babies who are nutritionally 'at risk' (e.g. when breastfed from a poorly nourished mother) should receive vitamins from the age of 1 month. Premature babies should have extra vitamins as soon as they start oral feeds. A suitable multivitamin preparation is Children's Vitamin Drops which contain vitamins A, C and D; the dose is 5 drops/day. An alternative is Abidec which contains vitamin B as well as A, C and D; the dose is 0.6 ml/day.

Once children stop receiving breast milk or formula milks, and go on to normal doorstep cow's milk (which is low in vitamins A and D) they should all start taking one of the vitamin preparations mentioned above. This is usually recommended until they are at least 2 years old, and preferably 5 years, depending on the rest of the diet. The current Department of Health recommendations are to give vitamins to all infants from the age of 6 months.

Iron supplementation is not necessary for breast- or bottle-fed babies. It should be given to premature babies as the iron stores are all laid down in the last trimester of pregnancy. They should start it after 2 weeks (if they are having oral feeds) and continue until they are 6 months old and on a normal mixed diet. Babies who are exclusively breastfed for more than 6 months, or who receive mainly cow's milk with no solids, will need extra iron as they will have depleted their own stores.

WEANING

Very few infants require solids before the age of 3 months, and most start around 4 months. They should all be on a mixed diet by 6 months. Some cultures delay weaning and give an exclusive milk diet (usually breast milk) even up to a year or more. This results in iron-deficiency anaemia and can also lead to behavioral feeding problems.

First solids tend to be cereals, rusks or commercial weaning foods. Ground rice should be the only cereal given for the first few months. It is recommended that gluten is not given before 4–6 months and eggs not before 9–12 months, especially in atopic families. Doorstep cow's milk is not advisable before 6 months. Full-cream milk should be used as skimmed and semi-skimmed milks are unsuitable until 5 years of age due to their lower energy and vitamin A and D content.

TUBE FEEDING

Feeding difficulties are frequently encountered in low birthweight babies. Premature babies less than 34 weeks gestation and babies under 2 kg usually have a poor sucking reflex. Assuming they are well enough to receive enteral feeds (i.e. into the gut), this will have to be administered through a nasogastric (NG) tube. Infants just above 2 kg may suck well but sometimes it is necessary to give a proportion of a feed or alternate feeds down a tube.

The tube is passed into the stomach via the nose. The usual distance is 20 cm but it should first be measured, from the tip of the nose to the external auditory meatus and then to the lower end of the sternum.

A PVC (Portex Blueline infant feeding) tube is used. Although larger babies can tolerate a size 8 FG tube, it is kinder to use a size 6 FG. Babies under 1 kg weight should have a size 4 FG.

The tube is passed by pushing it gently through the nostril and then directly backwards. It should easily curve downwards at the nasopharynx and then slide into the stomach. Failure to pass the tube should make you consider the possibility of a choanal atresia or if it is impeded further down an oesophageal atresia.

Fluid is aspirated and if it is colourless and gives a pink acid reaction on litmus paper then it is in the stomach. Another way of checking is to blow air down the tube whilst listening over the stomach with a stethoscope for the gurgling sounds. If green bilious fluid is withdrawn then you have gone through the pylorus and the tube should be withdrawn 2 cm and rechecked. Once the position is satisfactory, the tube is taped securely to the nose. Aspiration should be repeated before each feed is given to check it is still in the stomach and also to check whether the baby has retained the last feed rather than digested it. The tube should be replaced every 3 days.

At first the milk is given every hour or continuously via a syringe pump. If the baby tolerates this, it can then be given as a bolus feed, allowing gravity to let the milk run out of an open syringe, which is quicker than the pump. Once the feeds are well tolerated, if the BM stix are also satisfactory, the interval between feeds can gradually be increased and they will eventually be given every 3 hours. It may be preferable to give feeds continuously via a pump if the baby is very small as this avoids overdistending the stomach.

The daily milk requirement for a small baby is 60 ml/kg bodyweight/day on the first day increasing by 30 ml/kg/day. If the baby is having expressed breast milk or normal formula milk he can have up to 200 ml/kg/day. If he is on low birthweight formula milk then he should not go above 150 ml/kg/day unless weight gain is very poor.

Sometimes intrajejunal feeding is used in small babies. A radio-opaque silastic tube with a weighted end is used so that the position can be checked on X-ray. The tube is passed into the stomach and then should eventually pass through the pylorus with peristalsis. Milk is then given continuously via a pump. Its only real advantage is in babies who have severe gastro-oesophageal reflux or who are prone to frequent apnoeic episodes or vomiting. It may cause intestinal hurry and steatorrhoea by increasing the solute load in the small intestine and by reducing pancreatic enzyme secretion.

INTRAVENOUS FLUIDS

If a newborn baby is unwell it is usually safest not to feed the baby enterally. IV fluids will have to be administered through a small cannula into a peripheral vein (see p. 255). As the baby grows, the maintenance fluid requirement increases (Table 12.2).

If there are excessive losses (e.g. diarrhoea or vomiting) these must also be replaced. An additional 30 ml/kg/day is given if the baby is under phototherapy lights and a further 30 ml/kg/day if he is on an open incubator with an overhead heater.

Fullterm babies should be given 5% glucose whilst preterm babies are given 10% glucose. The glucose content may need to be altered depending on the blood glucose determined on the BM stix.

Table 12.2 Maintenance fluid requirement increases with age.

Age in days	Fullterm baby (ml/kg/day)	Preterm baby (ml/kg/day)
1	40	60
2	70	90
3	100	120
4	130	150
5 +	150	180

Maintenance sodium should be given from day one. From the second day, babies require potassium to be added to the fluids. Requirements are as follows:

sodium   2–3 mmol/kg/day;
potassium   2–3 mmol/kg/day.

The amounts may need to be varied according to the serum electrolytes.

The following is an example of how to calculate the fluids required for a typical fullterm baby who is a week old:

Weight of baby: 4 kg
Fluid requirement: 150 ml/kg/day of 5% glucose
                                    = 600 ml/day (i.e. 25 ml/hour).

Sodium and potassium
requirement: 2.5 mmol/kg/day = 10 mmol/day.

So the daily requirement of 600 ml of fluid must contain 10 mmol of sodium and potassium (i.e. a 500 ml bag of glucose must contain 8.3 mmol sodium and 8.3 mmol potassium).

The fluid chart should read as follows:

5% glucose 500 ml + 8 mmol NaCl
                            + 8 mmol KCl @ 25 ml/hour.

If a baby is receiving intravenous drugs but is feeding normally, in order to prevent the cannula from becoming blocked with a blood clot, it is best to run an infusion of 0.9% sodium chloride solution at 0.2 ml/hour from a syringe pump.

TOTAL PARENTERAL NUTRITION

Total parenteral nutrition (TPN) is a way of feeding a baby intravenously, usually via a centrally-placed catheter. The fluid used is a complex mixture of glucose, amino acids and lipids. It also contains all the necessary electrolytes, minerals and vitamins. The major role is in babies who are too sick to receive enteral feeds, as simple IV fluids do not contain enough calories to maintain the child for more than a few days. It is also used in babies who have severe gastrointestinal problems such as necrotizing enterocolitis or who have had bowel surgery. There is no advantage in giving TPN to low birthweight babies who are well enough to receive milk.

FURTHER READING

Department of Health and Social Security (1988) *Present Day Practice in Infant Feeding: Third Report.*DHSS Report on Health and Social Subjects 32. HMSO, London.
Levi J (1988) Establishing breast feeding in hospital. *Archives of Disease in Childhood*, **63**: 1281–5.
Martin J & White A (1988) *Infant Feeding 1985*. HMSO, London.

13: Vomiting

Vomiting is common in the newborn and most babies regurgitate to some degree. Although there is often nothing wrong, sometimes it is the only sign of an underlying serious illness. It is therefore most important to see the baby promptly and make a diagnosis.

The type of vomit and its relation to feeding may be most helpful. Types can be categorized as follows:
• frothy mucoid;
• bile-stained;
• blood-stained;
• milk.

FROTHY MUCOID 'VOMIT'

Oesophageal atresia with a tracheo-oesophageal fistula may present with vomiting, coughing and cyanosis when the infant begins the first feed. Vomiting of frothy mucoid material may be the only definite observation reported, but the condition should be suspected in any baby who has any symptoms during the first feed. It is not really vomit as it is not stomach contents but this is usually how it is described to the doctor. The management has been described on p. 105.

BILE-STAINED VOMIT

Bile-stained greenish yellow vomit in a baby is due to intestinal obstruction until proved otherwise. Until the diagnosis is confirmed this is an emergency as some of the causes need urgent treatment and surgical referral is mandatory.

Some forms of intestinal obstruction may present with vomiting of milk feeds before progressing to bile. Particular attention must be paid to the following points in the history and examination:
1 Is there abdominal distension?
2 Has any meconium been passed, and if so is it normal?
3 Is there an abdominal mass present?

Plain X-rays of the abdomen may be helpful by confirming the presence of obstruction. A supine and left lateral decubitus (the baby is lying on his left side) film is taken and obstruction is indicated by distended bowel with air–fluid levels. It is not usually possible to differentiate small from large bowel obstruction in the neonate on X-ray. Occasionally the X-ray is diagnostic (e.g. the 'double-bubble' of duodenal atresia or the intramural gas of necrotizing enterocolitis).

Whatever the cause, the initial management is the same. The child should be given maintenance IV fluids as outlined in the previous chapter. Added sodium and potassium will be necessary from the start. Serum electrolytes must be monitored at least twice a day and the IV fluids adjusted accordingly. Acid–base balance and blood glucose must also be checked.

The child must not be given oral fluids. A large nasogastric tube (size 8 FG) must be passed and kept on free drainage. Aspirates should be measured and replaced volume-for-volume by extra IV fluid consisting of 0.9% sodium chloride solution with 10 mmol KCl added to every 500-ml bag of fluid. Urine output should also be monitored and the child needs to be weighed daily. A very sick infant may need to be ventilated, and it is often safer to transfer the baby to the surgical referral centre on a ventilator.

If the mother can not travel with the baby, take 10 ml of her blood (clotted specimen) for crossmatching blood for the baby. She must also sign a consent form for the baby's laparotomy, and the parents should be informed that the baby may need a temporary colostomy.

Below are outlined some of the commoner causes of intestinal obstruction found in the neonate.

Duodenal atresia

The incidence is one in 6000 births and in 30% of cases it is associated with Down's syndrome. Obstruction is usually distal to where the common bile duct (CBD) enters the duodenum hence the cardinal sign of bile-stained vomiting. Abdominal distension is minimal but there may be visible peristalsis as well as infrequent passage of meconium. Diagnosis is usually confirmed by a plain abdominal X-ray which shows the 'double-bubble' sign of gaseous distension of the stomach and proximal duodenum in an abdomen with no other gas shadows. If the obstruction is proximal to the CBD there is no bile in the vomit and no abdominal distension so the diagnosis may be delayed. A one-stage anastomosis (duodeno-duodenostomy) is usually all that is needed.

Duodenal obstruction may not be complete, there may be stenosis or a web that partially obstructs the lumen. The duodenum may also be obstructed by extrinsic compression from peritoneal bands in a malrotated gut (see p. 150). With a partial intrinsic obstruction, there is often a delay in diagnosis. The vomiting may be bile-stained, but often contains milk as well, since the baby may be tolerating feeds. Meconium is usually passed and may even have progressed to the soft greenish brown changing stools. Plain X-ray may only show a mildly dilated stomach and duodenum so a barium meal may be necessary. Surgical removal of the obstruction will be necessary but is not an emergency.

Small bowel atresia

A low small intestinal obstruction presents within 48 hours with typical bile-stained vomiting, abdominal distension and failure to pass meconium. The baby may however pass small amounts of mucus which are occasionally stained with meconium. Distended loops of bowel are sometimes visible or palpable in the abdomen. X-ray shows dilated loops of bowel with air–fluid levels and an absence of bowel gas in the lower part of the abdomen. Sometimes there are multiple atresias connected by fibrous bands. Surgery is necessary to resect the area and perform an end-to-end anastomosis.

Malrotation

During early embryonic development, the intestine lies outside the abdominal cavity. When it returns, it should rotate into its normal position with the caecum in the right iliac fossa. Sometimes the rotation is incomplete which can have serious consequences. The caecum is in the right upper quadrant by the duodenum. Peritoneal (Ladds) bands may compress the second part of the duodenum causing a partial obstruction. The baby has intermittent bile-stained vomiting which eventually becomes persistent. The abdomen is not distended and the baby passes normal meconium. Plain X-ray is usually normal but barium studies of the upper bowel are usually diagnostic. The cardinal sign is the presence of the duodeno-jejunal (DJ) flexure to the right of the vertebral column (normally the duodenum crosses the midline and the DJ flexure is on the left side). Surgery consists simply of cutting through the Ladds bands which relieves the obstruction.

Malrotation with volvulus

Unfortunately malrotation sometimes leads to the serious complication of a midgut volvulus. The gut twists on the narrow-based mesentery and occludes its own blood supply. The baby becomes pale and the blood pressure falls. He may pass fresh blood per rectum or have a haematemesis. The plain X-ray usually shows an abdomen with no gas shadows. The baby needs vigorous resuscitation with colloid and an urgent surgical referral. This is an emergency since if the ischaemia is prolonged, the whole small intestine may infarct which can be fatal. Even if the child survives a major infarction, so much bowel may be lost that there is inadequate gut to sustain enteral feeding. There is as yet no place for gut transplantation and the child has to survive on long-term total parenteral nutrition.

Incarcerated inguinal hernia

The commonest time for an inguinal hernia to become incarcerated is in the newborn period. If the hernia becomes irreducible, the small intestine within it may strangulate. The screaming child presents with vomiting, abdominal distension and a red painful mass in the groin. Fortunately this is rarely seen now that inguinal herniae are repaired soon after diagnosis in babies. However, it highlights the importance of examining the groins of a baby who is vomiting.

Necrotizing enterocolitis (NEC)

This is usually seen in premature babies but outbreaks have been known to occur in previously well fullterm babies. The pathogenesis seems to involve ischaemic gut mucosa followed by infection with gas-forming organisms. Any part of the gut may be involved but the ileum and colon are most often affected. The exact aetiology is still unknown, but it is associated with prematurity, perinatal hypoxia, hypotension, respiratory distress syndrome, sepsis, exchange transfusions and umbilical vessel catheterization.

Early symptoms are non-specific, such as lethargy and poor feeding. This is followed by abdominal distension and the passage of fresh red blood in the stools. The abdomen becomes shiny and tender. The baby starts to vomit; this is milk at first but soon becomes bile-stained as the obstruction occurs. Sometimes faeculent vomiting ensues. The baby may have acidosis, hypothermia and hypotension. Periumbilical erythema and oedema of the abdominal wall are signs of intestinal necrosis and impending perforation. A sudden deterioration may indicate that the bowel has perforated.

Abdominal X-ray may be normal at first, but later may show pathognomonic intramural gas. The gas bubbles in the bowel wall produce a tramline appearance. Dilated bowel loops may be seen as well as air–fluid levels. In late stages, gas may be seen outlining the biliary tree in the liver. If the bowel has perforated, free gas will be seen under the diaphragm or at the upper side if a lateral decubitus X-ray is taken.

Conservative management is usually all that is needed. The child receives no oral fluid for 7–10 days and a NG tube is kept on free drainage. IV fluids are given and colloid if the child is hypotensive. Total parenteral nutrition will be necessary after 1–2 days. After taking blood cultures, IV antibiotics are necessary for 10 days (usually benzylpenicillin, gentamicin and metronidazole).

Perforation will require laparotomy which is extremely hazardous in these very sick babies. Sometimes excision of necrotic bowel is necessary in babies who show no improvement, but the decision when to operate can be very difficult. Some infants develop strictures with further obstruction as the gut heals after about 4 weeks. Mortality is still around 10% and rises to 25% if the bowel perforates.

Hirschsprung's disease

There is a congenital absence of ganglion cells in the wall of the distal part of the large bowel. The rectum is always involved and the disease extends proximally to a varying degree. The result is a functional intestinal obstruction at the level of the transition from normal to aganglionic bowel. It is commoner in boys and there is an association with Down's syndrome.

In the neonatal period, the disease presents either as delayed passage of meconium or complete intestinal obstruction. The best pointer to the diagnosis is failure to pass meconium within 48 hours. Abdominal distension soon ensues and there may be visible peristalsis in the epigastric region. The babies feed poorly and if complete obstruction follows, bile-stained vomiting is seen.

Always consider the diagnosis in any baby with delayed passage of meconium but first check whether the baby passed any at birth in case this has not been recorded. The first thing to do is a plain abdominal X-ray with the infant in an erect position. This will show classic signs of obstruction with dilated loops of bowel and air–fluid levels. It must be done before a rectal examination as this may relieve the obstruction and the X-ray may then be unhelpful.

The rectal examination itself is almost pathognomonic. The rectum is empty and feels tight. However it often induces a massive explosion of flatus which is followed by unending amounts of meconium once the finger is withdrawn.

Referral to a surgeon is necessary at this stage. A barium enema will be performed although ideally this is done before any rectal examination or at least not until 12–24 hours later, otherwise the true picture will be masked. It classically shows the narrow segment of aganglionic bowel widening out markedly as a cone of normal but distended bowel. Follow-up plain X-ray shows the barium is retained for over 24 hours.

The diagnosis is confirmed and the extent of the disease determined by a suction rectal biopsy and anorectal manometry (pressure studies). A relieving temporary colostomy will be necessary followed by definitive surgery after at least 4 months.

Occasionally the diagnosis is missed and an older child presents with abdominal distension, chronic severe constipation and a degree of malnutrition.

Another consequence of delayed diagnosis can be the serious complication of enterocolitis. The infant presents at 2–4 weeks with profuse bloody diarrhoea, marked abdominal distension and bile-stained vomiting. The child is usually extremely ill and may be in hypovolaemic shock.

Meconium ileus

This is the commonest way that children with cystic fibrosis (CF) present in the neonatal period; it occurs in 10–15% of all cases of CF. The meconium is thick, viscid and sticky hence the alternative name for CF of mucoviscidosis. The meconium impacts and obstructs the lumen of the ileum.

The presentation ranges from delayed passage of meconium to complete intestinal obstruction. In the latter cases, there is marked abdominal distension and bile-stained vomiting within 24 hours. As well as visible peristalsis, the loops of bowel can be palpated and feel as if they are full of putty.

There is a high rate of associated complications. There may be gangrenous bowel which can perforate, a volvulus (the heavy segment of bowel easily twists), atresia or meconium peritonitis.

In the latter, a perforation has occured *in utero* which has resealed. The meconium that escapes calcifies by birth.

Abdominal X-ray shows distended loops of bowel with a ground-glass appearance within the lumen due to air bubbles mixed with the meconium. There are usually no air–fluid levels unless there is a volvulus or atresia. Calcification in the peritoneal cavity implies meconium peritonitis. Free gas in the abdominal cavity is present if there is a perforation which is still open.

In uncomplicated cases, the obstruction can be treated conservatively. An enema of Gastrografin (X-ray contrast medium) is given that liquifies the meconium and facilitates its expulsion. Its very high osmolarity causes large amounts of fluid to be drawn into the gut so it is essential to keep the child well hydrated with extra IV fluid. If this fails to relieve the obstruction or there are signs of any complications, surgery will be necessary.

A sweat test is carried out to make the definitive diagnosis of cystic fibrosis but the collection of adequate volumes of sweat may be difficult before 3–4 weeks of age. In the meanwhile, an alternative method of diagnosis is to measure levels of immunoreactive trypsin (IRT) from a dried blood spot on a Guthrie card (see Appendix 6). Levels of IRT are elevated in CF, although after the age of 6 weeks, the IRT level may remain normal in a child with the disease.

Meconium plug
A single plug of inspissated meconium may cause a low intestinal obstruction. Rectal examination may cause the plug to be expelled and the obstruction is relieved. Sometimes a Gastrografin enema is necessary. Appropriate investigations must be performed to exclude Hirschsprung's disease and CF.

Obstruction with a palpable mass
Occasionally an abdominal mass is palpable in cases of intestinal obstruction. As outlined above, loops of bowel filled with thick meconium may be palpable in meconium ileus.

Duplications of the gut may also cause obstruction. This is a developmental abnormality in which part of the intestine, anywhere from the tongue to the anus, is duplicated. The duplication may be tubular or cystic. Tubular ones are uncommon and communicate with the intestinal lumen. Since they often contain gastric mucosa which causes peptic ulceration in adjacent normal bowel, they may present with bleeding or ulceration. The commoner cystic duplications are most often found in the small intestine where they cause obstruction, and are often palpable. Occasionally, they cause volvulus or an intussusception.

The mass may be extrinsic to the bowel but by compressing it causes obstruction. Examples would be tumours, such as a lymphoma, neuroblastoma or a nephroblastoma which can present, albeit rarely, in the newborn. A large hydronephrosis can also obstruct the bowel.

Functional obstruction
There are several causes of non-mechanical intestinal obstruction that lead to bile-stained vomiting and abdominal distension. These are relatively easy to differentiate from mechanical causes due to the presence of other relevant symptoms. In addition, although the X-ray will show widespread distension of the bowel, there are not usually air–fluid levels. Causes of paralytic ileus include:
- septicaemia;
- early necrotizing enterocolitis;
- birth asphyxia;
- respiratory distress syndrome;
- severe haemolytic disease of the newborn;
- hyponatraemia or hypokalaemia;
- functional immaturity of the bowel in premature babies;
- any very sick neonate.

BLOOD-STAINED VOMIT

Blood in the vomit is always alarming for parents. However it is only significant if macroscopic blood can be seen and even then the causes are often not serious. Nearly all vomit will test positive with Labstix to the minute amounts of blood that are normally produced by the act of vomiting, so it is pointless to routinely test vomit for blood.

Swallowed maternal blood
Maternal blood may be swallowed before delivery following premature separation of the placenta at birth. It also occurs quite commonly if the mother has cracked nipples and is breastfeeding the baby. If there is doubt over the diagnosis, maternal haemoglobin can be recognized in the vomit by the ability of alkali to denature it (APT's test).

Trauma
A nasogastric feeding tube frequently scratches the gastric mucosa and produces a few specks of blood in the vomit.

Haemorrhagic disease of the newborn
This is rarely seen now that babies are routinely given prophylactic vitamin K at birth. However it can occur if the dose was omitted and the baby is breastfeeding, as breast milk is deficient in vitamin K. The baby usually presents between the second and fourth day or, rarely, a few weeks after birth with haematemesis or melaena. If profuse, the child may become hypotensive and shocked. Treatment is to give vitamin K 1 mg IV, and fresh frozen plasma (which replaces several clotting factors) if necessary. The child may need a transfusion of fresh packed red cells, and in an emergency uncross-matched O-negative blood can be used.

Volvulus
Volvulus of the small intestine may lead to vomiting of dark red blood, but other signs will be present.

Hiatus hernia
Hiatus hernia with the complication of reflux oesophagitis can lead to persistent vomiting which is often blood-stained. Aspiration pneumonia and apnoeic episodes are other symptoms in the newborn.

MILK VOMIT

Infection
Infection commonly makes babies vomit their feeds. The

causes include:
- gastroenteritis which is rare in breastfed babies. Vomiting may precede diarrhoea for as long as 48 hours;
- urinary tract infection. Vomiting is often the only symptom (see p. 192);
- meningitis which causes vomiting due to cerebral irritation (see p. 187);
- septicaemia which must be excluded in any baby who is vomiting (see p. 186).

Feeding difficulties
This is one of the commonest causes of vomiting in the newborn. A ravenous infant may swallow excessive air at the beginning of a feed, and if the infant is not properly 'winded', milk may be regurgitated later with air. For further management see p. 137.

Gastro-oesophageal reflux
Gastro-oesophageal reflux (GOR) is usually associated with a sliding hiatus hernia but it can occur without any herniation, particularly in infants. In the first 3 months of life, the functional gastro-oesophageal sphincter is relatively weak. With increasing age, the lower oesophageal sphincter pressure increases and oesophageal motility becomes more organized. In addition, relatively more of the oesophagus comes to be situated within the abdomen. This explains why young babies can be 'burped' easily and why posseting, which is the regurgitation of small amounts of curdled milk, is so common. Because of the low acidity of the gastric juices in the first few months, the oesophageal mucosa is rarely damaged.

Reflux occurs readily and it can take the form of severe persistent vomiting. The vomiting starts in the first week and occurs soon after feeds in an effortless way. The vomit usually contains only milk but occasionally is streaked with blood. Severe reflux can be associated with failure to thrive, and recurrent aspiration pneumonia with recurrent bronchospasm. It can eventually lead to oesophageal ulceration, stricture formation and dysphagia.

Diagnosis is best confirmed by 24-hour pH monitoring of the lower oesophagus. A probe the size of a nasogastric tube is placed just above the gastro-oesophageal sphincter. It records the pH and the results are analysed on a computer. If this is not available, a barium swallow may be helpful but a normal study does not exclude GOR. An alternative test is a milk scan in which the baby is fed milk which contains a radioisotope which can be viewed on a gamma camera. Oesophagoscopy may also be necessary.

Minor degrees of GOR recover spontaneously, usually within the first year, but this is not much consolation to the mother who has vomit permanently down her back.

It should be said that most babies do not need any treatment, and conservative measures should be tried first. The milk can be thickened by adding agents such as Carobel. The child should sleep prone with the mattress angled so his head is higher than his feet. Mild antacids may help, although Gaviscon should not be used in infants under 6 months due to the high sodium content. The new drug cisapride increases the tone of the lower oesophageal sphincter and reduces GOR but is not yet licensed for young children.

In rare cases, surgery is required. A Nissen's fundoplication is performed and although this usually abolishes reflux, it must be noted that the children can no longer vomit which can be misleading if they subsequently develop intestinal obstruction.

Intestinal obstruction
All forms of obstruction may start with vomiting of milk before becoming bile stained.

High duodenal obstruction presents with vomiting of milk without bile if the lesion is proximal to the entrance of the common bile duct into the duodenum.

Pyloric stenosis is a common condition but does not usually present in the newborn. It tends to occur between 2–6 weeks and is much commoner in baby boys. The hallmark is effortless projectile vomiting which resembles a fountain and can travel several feet. The baby is unperturbed but may become chronically hungry. The classic picture of a dehydrated malnourished infant is rarely seen nowadays.

Diagnosis is made by palpating the pyloric tumour during a test feed. Wear an apron and sit on the baby's left side. While the mother feeds the child (breast or bottle), palpate the abdomen. The tumour is the size of the tip of your little finger and feels very hard. It is felt adjacent to the lateral edge of the right rectus abdominis muscle just below the ribs. The tumour 'comes and goes' and is best felt just after the baby has vomited. Sometimes it is immediately obvious but the test feed may have to be repeated several times before you are convinced. In 10–20% of cases the tumour is impalpable. Visible peristalsis of the stomach may sometimes be seen. The diagnosis can be confirmed with an ultrasound examination. If there is still doubt, a barium meal is performed.

Venous pH should be checked. It is usually alkalotic with a slightly raised bicarbonate (25–30 mmol/l). Serum electrolytes should also be checked.

Once confirmed, the child should receive IV fluids and nothing orally. Ensure the baby received vitamin K at birth, and if there is any doubt this should be given. The child will need surgery but this is not an emergency and should only be performed once acid–base balance and serum electrolytes are normal. The operation is a Ramstedt's pyloromyotomy in which the outer muscle coat of the pylorus is divided down to the mucosa.

As long as the mucosa is not breached at operation, the babies can restart milk 12 hours after surgery. If bottle fed, some people advocate starting on diluted milk. There is no point starting on water or glucose as if the child vomits it is safer if the stomach contents are buffered by milk.

Milk plug syndrome can occur in small babies who are receiving large volumes of formula milk to prevent hypoglycaemia. Thick milk curds may obstruct the pylorus causing abdominal distension and vomiting. A gastric washout is necessary followed by gradually increasing strengths of milk. Occasionally the milk blocks the small intestine after the fourth day and the child develops intestinal obstruction with a picture similar to meconium ileus. This is not seen in breastfed babies.

OTHER RARE CAUSES

1 Raised intracranial pressure due for example to intracranial haemorrhage.

2 Drugs, especially digoxin.

3 Congenital adrenal hyperplasia (see p. 111) commonly presents with vomiting as the only symptom in the male, but this is not usually for the first 10 days.

4 Metabolic diseases, for example galactosaemia or urea cycle disorders.

FURTHER READING

Milla PJ & Muller DPR (1988) *Harries' Paediatric Gastroenterology.* Churchill Livingstone, Edinburgh.

Spitz L, Steiner GM & Zachary RB (1989) *A Colour Atlas of Paediatric Surgical Diagnosis.* Wolfe Medical Publications Ltd, London.

14: Hypoglycaemia

A lack of glucose is as devastating to the brain as a lack of oxygen. Hypoglycaemia is an emergency and must be treated promptly.

DEFINITION

Significant hypoglycaemia is said to occur in term babies with a plasma glucose <1.9 mmol/l during the first 72 hours and <2.6 mmol/l after this period. In premature and small-for-dates babies, the cut-off is set at 1.4 mmol/l.

Some authorities would accept a plasma glucose level down to 1.6 mmol/l in term babies and 1.1 mmol/l in low birthweight babies. This is a controversial issue but it seems sensible to opt for the higher safety margin.

CAUSES

1 *Small-for-date babies* who have suffered from intrauterine growth retardation have reduced glycogen and fat stores.

2 *Preterm babies* also have a lack of glycogen reserves as these are primarily laid down in the last 4 weeks of pregnancy.

3 *Infants of diabetic mothers (IDM)* usually have a raised blood glucose throughout the pregnancy, depending on the level of control of the mother's diabetes. This leads to pancreatic islet-cell hyperplasia so that the IDM is hyperinsulinaemic. Once the baby is born and cut off from the rich source of maternal glucose, the baby rapidly becomes hypoglycaemic due to the high levels of circulating insulin. The blood glucose drops in the first 1–2 hours, sometimes to less than 1 mmol/l, but normally starts to rise again at 3–4 hours.

4 *Poor feeding* may sometimes lead to hypoglycaemia. This is unusual but can occur in breastfed babies after 3 or 4 days of poor intake.

5 *Severe birth asphyxia* leads to hypoglycaemia as the liver and heart become depleted of glycogen.

6 *Sick babies* are prone to hypoglycaemia if the illness is severe, for example in septicaemia or congenital heart disease. Hypoglycaemia is often associated with hypothermia, due to increased metabolic rate. Conversely, sometimes the stress of severe illness causes a raised blood glucose due to the release of catecholamines, glucagon and cortisol.

7 *Haemolytic disease of the newborn* also results in islet-cell hyperplasia and hyperinsulinism. The severity is related to the severity of the anaemia. An exchange transfusion may also lead to hypoglycaemia.

8 *Polycythaemia* may be associated with hypoglycaemia.

9 *Rare causes* should be considered in cases where the hypoglycaemia is persistent and difficult to control. There are several inborn disorders of carbohydrate metabolism (e.g. glycogen storage disease, galactosaemia) and amino acid metabolism (e.g. maple syrup urine disease, propionic acidaemia and tyrosinosis). Beckwith–Wiedemann syndrome (exomphalos, macroglossia, gigantism) is associated with islet-cell hyperplasia and hypoglycaemia occurs in up to half the cases. Islet-cell adenomas and nesidioblastosis also cause hyperinsulinism. Endocrine disorders (e.g. anterior pituitary, adrenal or thyroid gland) can also lead to hypoglycaemia.

SYMPTOMS

Hypoglycaemia is often asymptomatic and may only then be detected by performing a BM stix test for blood glucose.

Symptoms that are most often associated with hypoglycaemia include:

- recurrent apnoea;
- vomiting;
- jitteriness;
- convulsions.

It is most important that any baby that has a convulsion has an immediate BM stix measurement.

The classic symptoms seen in older children and adults due to catecholamine release (pallor, sweating, tachycardia and faintness) are not seen in neonates unless there is severe hyperinsulinism.

MANAGEMENT

Prevention

Management is primarily aimed at prevention. High-risk groups need to be identified and have their blood glucose monitored regularly at first. This can be done with a heel-prick capillary sample using the BM stix test. If the BM reads <1.4 mmol/l, a venous blood sample should be taken to measure the true plasma glucose.

The key to prevention is early feeding. Small-for-dates babies should start milk feeds within 2 hours of birth and be fed 3-hourly for the first 24 hours. They should be able to suck normally but if there is a problem then the milk is given via a nasogastric (NG) tube. Regular BM stix can be discontinued once they are consistently above 2 mmol/l for 24 hours, as long as the baby is feeding well.

Premature babies who are unwell, or who are likely to develop respiratory problems due to their gestational age, should not be given enteral feeds initially. They should have an IV line inserted without delay and a 10% glucose infusion started with maintenance sodium.

IDM babies should also start early feeds within 1–2 hours, using a NG tube if necessary. They should be fed 3-hourly for the first 24 hours. If they are to be bottle fed, they should be given 60 ml/kg/day. Breastfed babies should be put to the breast but may need complementary formula milk if the glucose falls below 1.5 mmol/l. IV glucose should be avoided if at all possible as the high glucose load exacerbates the hyperinsulinism, whereas glucose is absorbed more slowly through the stomach and does not lead to such a marked insulin surge.

A BM stix should be done in the labour ward shortly after birth as hypoglycaemia may even be present this early. BM stix should then be performed 2-hourly for the first 12 hours or before each feed, and can then be discontinued if the blood glucose is normal and the baby is feeding well.

All asphyxiated and sick babies will be on IV infusions of glucose but should have the blood glucose monitored every 4–6 hours.

Treatment of asymptomatic hypoglycaemia

As soon as a low BM stix is noted, the baby should be given the next feed that is due. If he will not take the milk, then it must be given down a NG tube. In a breastfed baby, if there is no breast milk available, a single feed of 5% glucose may be given.

Repeat the BM stix, 1 hour after this feed. If it is still low, a venous blood sample should be taken which can be done at the same time as inserting an IV cannula.

A bolus of IV glucose should then be given. In hyperinsulinaemic babies (e.g. IDM), it is best to use 10% glucose as higher concentrations make rebound hypoglycaemia more likely. A bolus of 0.5 g/kg is given which is 5 ml/kg of 10% glucose (remember, a 10% solution contains 10 g/100 ml).

After the bolus is given, an infusion of 10% glucose should start at 60 ml/kg/day in all cases. A repeat bolus may be necessary, depending on the initial response, and occasionally a 15 or 20% glucose infusion is necessary. At the same time, milk should continue, either orally or via a NG tube. The slower absorption of glucose through the stomach will lessen the chances of rebound hypoglycaemia. A careful check of fluid volumes must be kept in order that the baby is not overloaded.

The IV glucose can normally be tailed off over 24 hours, and the BM stix should be checked 3-hourly over this period.

Treatment of symptomatic hypoglycaemia

Treatment is similar to the above scheme except that the IV bolus of glucose is given immediately followed by the IV infusion. Anticonvulsant drugs are not necessary and fitting will cease once the glucose is normal.

If it is not possible to insert an IV cannula immediately, an interim measure is to give an intramuscular injection of 250 µg glucagon.

LONG-TERM EFFECTS

The neonatal brain has the capacity to utilize alternative sources of fuel such as ketones and lactate. This means that low blood sugar has less effect on the neonatal brain than the adult brain. However, if the hypoglycaemia is prolonged and particularly if it is associated with convulsions or apnoea, there may be severe neurological sequelae. Up to a third of these babies develop serious developmental abnormalities including cerebral palsy and severe mental retardation.

It has also recently been realized that moderate asymptomatic hypoglycaemia is not as harmless as previously thought, and can also lead to neurodevelopmental impairment.

15: Jaundice

DEFINITION

Jaundice is a yellow discoloration of the skin due to the deposition of bilirubin pigment. This occurs when the serum bilirubin is raised.

PATHOPHYSIOLOGY

Red cell breakdown

| releases haemoglobin which
is broken down and then
the haem is metabolized to

Unconjugated bilirubin
(fat-soluble and bound to serum albumin)

| this is conjugated in the
liver by the glucuronyl
transferase enzymes

Conjugated bilirubin
(water-soluble)

| this is excreted from the
liver into the gut

Bile

In general, a rise in unconjugated bilirubin is due to pre-hepatic causes. It occurs when there is an increased breakdown of the red blood cells (haemolysis), which exceeds the conjugating capacity of the liver. When the problem lies in the liver or its conjugating enzymes, there is usually a mixed picture of raised unconjugated and conjugated bilirubin. A predominant rise in conjugated bilirubin is usually due to interference with excretion of the bilirubin into the bile after conjugation. This will eventually be accompanied by a rise in unconjugated bilirubin.

Conjugated hyperbilirubinaemia is *always* pathological in neonates and must be fully investigated.

CAUSES

Physiological
Jaundice due to a functional immaturity of the liver and its enzymes is particularly common in preterm infants. It also occurs frequently in term babies. A temporary deficiency of glucuronyl transferases reduces the rate of conjugation of bilirubin with a consequent rise in unconjugated bilirubin. In addition, there is a rapid haemolysis of fetal red cells that takes places after birth.

In fullterm infants, jaundice appears after the first 24 hours following birth, and reaches a peak on the fourth or fifth day. The changes in serum bilirubin precede the visible jaundice so that serum levels peak on the third day, drop rapidly by day 6 and are normal by 11–14 days. In preterm babies the jaundice usually begins within 48 hours of birth, and may last up to 2 weeks.

Breastfeeding
Breastfeeding is associated with jaundice due to elevated unconjugated bilirubin levels. There seem to be two separate types of breast milk jaundice. The early type occurs in the first 5 days and seems to be an exaggerated form of physiological jaundice. It is often attributed to poor fluid intake in the early stages of breastfeeding but there is really no evidence to confirm this.

The late type is recognized towards the end of the first week and usually continues for 3–6 weeks, and sometimes even 2–3 months. It is a diagnosis of exclusion and by definition the babies are otherwise completely healthy. There are theories that it is due to the presence of progesterone metabolites or free fatty acids in the milk but the evidence is inconclusive.

If breastfeeding is stopped and formula milk given for 48 hours, there is a rapid fall in bilirubin level. In the meanwhile the mother should express her milk otherwise lactation may cease. When breast milk is restarted, the bilirubin rises a little (usually by 20–60 μmol/l) but never again to the previously high level.

Red cell incompatibility
Jaundice is usually of rapid onset and is noted within the first 24 hours after birth. The incompatibility leads to haemolysis of red

blood cells causing an unconjugated hyperbilirubinaemia. There are different types:

1 *Rhesus incompatibility.* The mother is rhesus-negative while the infant is rhesus-positive. This condition is dealt with on p. 26.

2 *ABO incompatibility.* The mother's blood is group O and the infant's group A, or less commonly group B. Unlike rhesus incompatibility this can affect a first baby. The jaundice is less severe than with rhesus disease.

3 *Other blood groups* such as C, c, E, e, Kell and Duffy can also cause haemolytic jaundice.

Increased red cell breakdown

The system of normal conjugation can be overloaded and this results in an unconjugated hyperbilirubinaemia. A traumatic delivery that leads to extensive bruising will inevitably produce jaundice and preterm babies are particularly susceptible to this. A cephalhaematoma (see p. 70) always causes jaundice when the blood clot is broken down.

If the baby is polycythaemic and appears very red on the first day, the mother can be warned that he will soon turn yellow as the extra red cell load is broken down.

Infection

1 *Septicaemia* will result in jaundice due to increased red cell destruction, but this is usually of slightly later onset, around 3–4 days. The child will appear ill and there will usually be other symptoms and signs.

2 *Urinary tract infection* can present with jaundice which may be the only sign.

3 *Viral hepatitis* due to intrauterine infection with CMV, rubella or toxoplasma can result in early jaundice if the baby is severely affected. Occasionally hepatitis B will cause early severe jaundice and liver failure (see p. 21). There are pale stools and dark urine and the serum bilirubin is mainly conjugated.

Rare causes

1 *Biliary atresia* is a condition in which the bile ducts, both inside and outside the liver, become blocked due to a progressive inflammatory reaction. This leads to a severe obstructive conjugated jaundice, and if untreated biliary cirrhosis ensues and the infant dies within a year. Surgical correction is possible but only has a good chance of success if it is done by 8–9 weeks of age. The later alternative is a liver transplant which is far more hazardous than corrective surgery. We must emphasize the importance of proper investigation of infants with prolonged jaundice, particularly if there is an obstructive pattern. These infants are normally perfectly well for the first 4–8 weeks of life apart from mild jaundice. However, suspicion must be aroused if the urine is dark (yellow as opposed to clear or colourless) and the stools pale (containing no yellow or green pigment) or there is a conjugated hyperbilirubinaemia. Prompt referral to a specialist centre is then crucial.

2 *Hypothyroidism* causes a prolonged conjugated and unconjugated jaundice but the mechanism is not understood.

3 *Galactosaemia* is a rare autosomal recessive condition in which there is a deficiency of the enzyme responsible for the conversion of galactose to glucose. Galactose is one of the monosaccharide constituents of lactose which is the principle sugar found in milk. Prolonged conjugated jaundice and hepatosplenomegaly is one of the presentations. Other features are septicaemia, vomiting, hypotonia, lethargy, poor weight gain, and occasionally cataracts. The urine should be tested for reducing substances with the Clinitest which is positive in galactosaemia, and also Clinistix which tests for glucose and so will be negative. Diagnosis is confirmed by enzyme assays on red blood cells. In the meanwhile the infants must be fed on a lactose-free milk such as Galactomin. The importance of early diagnosis is that this is a preventable cause of mental retardation.

4 *Glucose-6-phosphate dehydrogenase (G6PD) deficiency* affects infants of Mediterranean, Middle Eastern, African and Far Eastern origin. It is an X-linked condition in which there is a deficiency of the enzyme responsible for maintaining the stability of the red blood cell membrane. In the neonate it usually presents with a severe unconjugated jaundice. It may also present with an attack of acute haemolysis or later with a chronic haemolytic anaemia.

G6PD levels can be measured in the blood.

The haemolytic episodes in babies can occur without the usual precipitating factors of drugs or infection. However the parents should be given a list of drugs that the child must avoid (see *British National Formulary*). The commonest one are aspirin, chloroquine, high doses of vitamin C, diphenhydramine which is present in Benylin and other cold remedies, co-trimoxazole, chloramphenicol, nalidixic acid and nitrofurnatoin. Eating broad (fava) beans, and fumes from mothballs can also precipitate an attack.

5 α_1-*antitrypsin deficiency* is a major cause of liver disease in children. It may present early as prolonged obstructive jaundice with raised levels of conjugated bilirubin. This may be accompanied by irritability, lethargy and failure to thrive. It is difficult to differentiate clinically from biliary atresia but blood levels of α_1-antitrypsin can be measured. There is no specific treatment although liver transplant remains an option.

Associated conditions

There are several conditions which are often associated with jaundice, although are not necessarily causally-linked. These include pyloric stenosis and high intestinal obstructions, Down's syndrome and Turner's syndrome, infants of diabetic mothers and cystic fibrosis.

EFFECTS

High levels of fat-soluble unconjugated bilirubin can damage brain cells in the basal ganglia and brain stem. This results in kernicterus and bilirubin encephalopathy. Acutely there may may be stupor, hypertonia, tremors or convulsions and fever. If severe, the condition may be fatal. The chronic neurological sequelae include athetoid cerebral palsy and deafness. Kernicterus is more likely to follow rhesus incompatibility than other causes of jaundice. Preterm babies are particularly susceptible to kernicterus and can develop it at lower bilirubin levels than fullterm babies. High levels of conjugated bilirubin do not have these effects.

Recent evidence has shown that neurological problems are most unlikely at serum bilirubin levels <170 μmol/l, even in babies weighing less than 1250 g. Whilst neurological impairment has been associated with levels >340 μmol/l, the risk of brain damage is very small in healthy fullterm infants unless levels reach at least 400–425 μmol/l.

ASSESSING SEVERITY

Clinically

The severity of jaundice can be assessed by skin colour, although this should only be used as a rough guide. Clearly it can be misleading in dark-skinned Asian and Afro-Caribbean babies but in these babies the colour of the sclerae can be helpful, as can the colour of palms and soles.

The yellow colour begins in the face, then proceeds down to the trunk and then to the limbs and finally the palms and soles. The point of most distal progression is assessed by pressing on the skin with your thumb to make it blanch and seeing whether it appears yellow. It can be misleading if light reflects off yellow or orange curtains and bedspreads and it is best to look at the skin colour under natural or fluorescent lighting.

Jaundice is not usually noticed at serum bilirubin levels less than 70 μmol/l. Table 15.1 is a guide to assessing bilirubin levels in fullterm babies — see also Fig. 15.1.

A useful device that midwives and general practitioners can use to assess jaundice at home is the icterometer. It is a piece of clear plastic which is pressed against the baby's nose. The colour

Table 15.1 Guide to assessing bilirubin levels in fullterm babies.

Location on baby	Serum bilirubin levels (μmol/l)
Face only	100
Trunk	150
Lower abdomen and thighs	200
Arms and lower legs	250
Hands and feet	>270

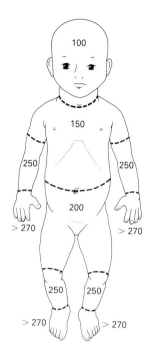

Fig. 15.1 Estimate of serum bilirubin (μmol/l) obtained by assessing distal progression of jaundice. Adapted from Kramer LI (1969) Advancement of dermal icterus in the jaundiced newborn. *American Journal of Diseases of Children*, **118**: 454–8.

of the tip of the nose is compared to five coloured strips on the plastic. This gives a guide to the level of jaundice and an indication when blood should be taken.

A clinical assessment of the baby's health should always be carried out. Particular attention should be paid to lethargy, floppiness and how well the baby is feeding. The colour of urine and stools should be checked, and this can usually be done by simply looking at the nappy. An obstructive cause is suggested by dark urine (normally it is clear or colourless) and pale stools for 2–3 days.

Blood tests

The serum bilirubin is the key to assessing the severity of jaundice. All that is needed is a small capillary blood sample taken from a heel-prick. This is centrifuged for a few minutes and easily read in a bilirubinometer which most paediatric departments possess. It is advisable to take a spare capillary sample as the tubes often disintegrate in the centrifuge. The samples should not be left in the light if there is a delay before processing them as the bilirubin is degraded and you will get a falsely low result. The machine gives the total bilirubin (unconjugated and conjugated) but this is enough for initial assessment of severity and for monitoring treatment. Alternatively, a sample of venous blood (0.5 ml in orange lithium heparin bottle) can be sent to the laboratory. In this case, the conjugated and unconjugated fractions will also be obtained.

The level of serum bilirubin that is acceptable depends on the age of the child and whether the baby is premature or full term. Charts exist for different gestational ages that give a guidance to the necessity for treatment (phototherapy charts) and these are outlined in Appendix 5. Values should always be plotted on these charts as it is the rate of the rise over the first few days that give the best indication over what action is necessary.

INVESTIGATING THE CAUSE

The investigations carried out depend on the timing of the jaundice as this gives a clue to the most likely aetiology.

1 *Onset within first 24 hours — whatever the level.* The diagnosis is probably a blood group incompatibility so carry out the following:
- serum bilirubin — both conjugated and unconjugated;
- full blood count and blood film;
- blood group; ⎱
- Coombs' test ⎰   0.5 ml of clotted blood.

2 *Onset after 24 hours but serum bilirubin >300 μmol/l.* Babies with mild jaundice who are perfectly well, need only have the serum bilirubin monitored and can be assumed to have physiological jaundice. However if the bilirubinometer result is high enough to suggest that the baby requires phototherapy, even if the baby is asymptomatic, the causes of the jaundice should be investigated as follows:
- serum bilirubin — conjugated and unconjugated;
- full blood count and white count differential;
- blood group;

- Coombs' test;
- blood culture (for latent infection);
- urine culture (for asymptomatic infection);
- G6PD levels in the appropriate racial groups (0.5 ml blood in a pink EDTA bottle).

3 *Prolonged jaundice >14 days.*
- serum bilirubin — conjugated and unconjugated;
- full blood count and differential;
- thyroid function tests;
- liver enzymes;
- G6PD if appropriate;
- urine culture;
- urine for reducing substances (for galactosaemia);
- urine for presence of bilirubin which reflects a high conjugated bilirubin (on a Labstix).

NB: In all cases of conjugated hyperbilirubinaemia or obstructive jaundice, biliary atresia must be excluded.

TREATMENT

Phototherapy

The serum bilirubin result should be plotted on a phototherapy chart (see Appendix 5). The charts indicate levels above which phototherapy is necessary. If the result is well below the line, no further action is necessary but the child should be reassessed the next day. If the jaundice has deepened then another serum bilirubin should be measured.

In a fullterm baby, after the fifth day, a serum bilirubin of 320 μmol/l is the cut-off for phototherapy. Up to 5 days, the acceptable level depends on the age of the infant. In preterm babies the cut-off for treatment is reduced, so for example babies born at 34–37 weeks should have phototherapy if the SBR is >270 μmol/l. There are phototherapy charts for the different gestational ages. Phototherapy is ineffective at levels below 100 μmol/l.

The serum bilirubin rises in a linear fashion, so if the value is just below the line, it should be repeated within 8 hours, as by then it may be high enough to necessitate treatment. If it remains below but parallel to the line then phototherapy is not necessary.

Almost all babies with a high serum bilirubin can be successfully treated with phototherapy, and some modern phototherapy units are very effective. Treatment consists of shining a 'blue' light on to the baby's skin. In some machines the light appears white but it is still at the appropriate wavelength. The light is not ultraviolet despite popular myth. It works by metabolizing and degrading the unconjugated bilirubin in the skin. This reduces the serum levels as more bilirubin then enters the skin and is in turn degraded.

When phototherapy is started, the serum bilirubin should be checked twice a day. Once it begins to fall or at least levels off, the phototherapy can stop. The SBR should then be rechecked 12–24 hours later. Sometimes phototherapy needs to be recommenced.

Probably the greatest drawback to phototherapy is the anxiety it provokes in the parents. This can be lessened by a careful explanation and treatment can take place on the postnatal ward beside the mother; there is no need to separate the mother from her baby.

The baby should be completely undressed, including no nappy, to maximize the area of skin exposed to the light. This means there is a risk of the baby getting cold and so the temperature should be checked every 3–4 hours. The room must be kept warm enough. Sometimes a perspex heat shield is necessary to help prevent heat loss. Conversely, care must be taken not to overheat the baby.

The baby should wear eye pads to protect the eyes from the bright light and these should not be too tight. The eye pads are thrown away after use and should never be reused for another baby.

Under the phototherapy lights, there is increased water loss through the skin. This is particularly so in premature babies with their thin skin so they should receive an extra 30 ml/kg/day of fluid. As long as a fullterm baby is feeding well, extra fluid is not necessary. If breastfeeding is not well established or the baby has diarrhoea (which sometimes occurs with phototherapy due to decreased gut transit time) then extra water can be given.

Recently there has been a trend to send babies home from the postnatal ward after only 1–2 days. This is often before significant jaundice has appeared. However the community midwife has the responsibility to check the baby for 10 days and should notice any developing jaundice. She can use an icterometer and if necessary take a heel-prick blood sample to have the serum bilirubin checked in the hospital. Occasionally babies have to be readmitted to hospital for phototherapy and this is always very upsetting for the parents.

Exchange transfusion
Occasionally phototherapy is not sufficient to combat an ever-increasing bilirubin level. This rarely happens now due to the low incidence of severe rhesus incompatibility resulting from the preventive measures undertaken with rhesus-negative mothers. In addition the modern phototherapy units work very efficiently. Sometimes double phototherapy, in which two lamps are used, is needed to keep the serum bilirubin down.

If the bilirubin is still rising, an exchange transfusion may be necessary. The phototherapy charts give guidelines for when to give an exchange transfusion but these are on the cautious side and there is a certain amount of leeway in healthy fullterm babies. Each case must be considered individually and the decision should be made by a senior paediatrician.

The main indications are in cases of severe jaundice due to haemolytic disease of the newborn. In addition to lowering the serum bilirubin it removes some of the haemolytic antibodies and corrects anaemia. It acts quickly so that it is useful in babies who are showing early signs of bilirubin encephalopathy.

The principal is to completely exchange the baby's blood with donor blood. Obviously this can not be done in one stage so a small amount is withdrawn which is followed by transfusion of an equal amount. This cycle is then repeated many times until enough blood has been exchanged. For a complete exchange twice the baby's blood volume is used (i.e. 170 ml/kg body-weight).

An exchange transfusion is hazardous although a scrupulously careful technique will lessen the risks.

POLYCYTHAEMIA

This is included in this chapter as polycythaemia leads to jaundice and its treatment is also by exchange transfusion.

Definition

Polycythaemia is essentially having too many red blood cells in the circulation. It is defined as a haematocrit (HCt) greater than 65% in a venous blood sample or 70% in a heel-prick capillary sample. A capillary sample that is high must always be confirmed with a venous (or arterial) sample. The HCt is calculated by centrifuging the sample in a capillary tube for at least 10 minutes, then measuring the proportion of red cells to plasma. This gives a slightly different result from the packed cell volume (PCV) calculated by the Coulter counter in the haematology laboratory. It is important to use either the HCt or the PCV but they should not be interchanged when monitoring progress.

Causes

1 Delayed clamping of the cord at delivery.
2 Recipient of a twin-to-twin transfusion.
3 Infants of diabetic mothers.
4 Intrauterine growth retardation.

Effects

The baby looks plethoric and very red. The problems lie in the fact that there is an increased blood viscosity with a high PCV which increases exponentially above 65%. This affects blood flow through the capillaries which may become rather sluggish.

The main risk is of cerebral venous thrombosis which can cause convulsions and damage to the brain. The cardiovascular system may also be affected and congestive cardiac failure or pulmonary hypertension can occur. There is an increased incidence of respiratory distress and transient tachypnoea of the newborn (Chapter 19). Jaundice always follows due to the large red cell load. Polycythaemia is also associated with hypoglycaemia and hypocalcaemia. Finally, due to the poor capillary flow there is an association with necrotizing enterocolitis and renal vein thrombosis.

Treatment

When to treat polycythaemia is controversial. Some would only treat symptomatic babies or those with a very high PCV (e.g. 80%). Alternatively, some treat all babies with a PCV >70%, with the idea that symptoms should be prevented. Since cerebral venous thrombosis can be devastating, and treatment is not difficult, we would favour the cautious approach.

Treatment involves a partial exchange transfusion using 20–30 ml/kg of plasma which dilutes the thickened blood. The method is otherwise similar to that used for jaundice. However it may be better to use peripheral lines only as this decreases the risks of the exchange transfusion. In this way the risk-benefit ratio favours treatment at a venous PCV of 70%.

FURTHER READING

Gartner LM & Auerbach KG (1987) Breast milk and breastfeeding jaundice. *Advances in Pediatrics*, **34**: 249–274.
Hussein M, Howard ER, Mieli-Vergani G & Mowat AP (1991) Jaundice at 14 days of age: exclude biliary atresia. *Archives of Disease in Childhood*, **66**: 1177–9.
Editorial (1991) Moderate neonatal hyperbilirubinaemia: hold tight. *Lancet* **338**: 1242–3.

16: Hot and Cold Babies

Babies normally maintain a temperature of 36.8–37°C with little variation. Fever is arbitrarily defined as a temperature above 37.5°C while hypothermia is a body temperature below 35°C.

Rectal temperatures are often taken and this must be done very carefully. It is sufficient to insert the thermometer 2 cm and it should never be inserted more than 3 cm as there is a risk of perforating the rectum, particularly in a struggling baby. Routine temperatures should be taken from the axilla and if abnormal, checked rectally. The skin temperature is normally 0.5–1°C lower than that in the rectum.

FEVER

Causes

Environmental temperature

Some infants, particularly those of low birthweight, have difficulty in maintaining a steady temperature and are susceptible to changes in the environmental temperature. The ideal temperature to nurse babies is that at which the oxygen consumption is lowest. This is known as thermoneutrality. It varies depending on the size of the baby (smaller babies need warmer temperatures); the age (as babies get older they do not need to be so warm) and on the amount of clothing worn. Neonatal units should be maintained at around 26–28°C to minimize heat loss from incubators. The recommended temperature for a baby's room at home is 18°C. If the room is too hot they can become pyrexial.

Babies can easily become overheated if put too near a radiator or fire, or if left in direct sunlight. Phototherapy can also heat the baby.

Overdressing

This is a common cause of a hot baby. For the first 4 weeks babies do need to be warmly dressed, but they should never be sweating nor feel hot to the touch. Feeling the baby's hands and feet can be misleading as these often feel cold; a better indication of whether the baby is hot or cold is to feel the trunk or abdomen.

Once a baby is over a month old, when they are indoors they need the same amount of clothes as their parents need to feel comfortable. When outdoors, they will need extra clothing but this must be removed as soon as they are taken back indoors, especially if there is central heating. This also applies if the baby is put into a car or a train.

When the babies are in a cot, they need no more than a nappy, vest and babygro. The amount of bedding depends on the room temperature although how hot the baby feels should also be taken into account (Table 16.1). Duvets are not recommended for infants less than 1 year old, nor should babies be covered by a sheepskin. Hot water bottles should also not be used.

Table 16.1 Amount of bedding needed by babies.

Room temperature	Amount of bedding
15°C (60°F)	Sheet + 4 layers of blankets
18°C (65°F)	Sheet + 3–4 layers of blankets
21°C (70°F)	Sheet + 2–3 layers of blankets
24°C (75°F)	Sheet + 1 layer of blanket
27°C (80°F)	Sheet only

Infection

If a baby is still pyrexial despite a normal environmental temperature and the right amount of clothing, then infection must always be considered. It should be remembered that a normal temperature does not exclude an infection, and in fact babies who are very unwell with sepsis are often hypothermic rather than febrile.

Likely infections in the newborn are:
• pneumonia;
• umbilical infection;
• septicaemia;
• meningitis;
• urinary tract infection;
• gastroenteritis.

A full infection screen should be carried out as outlined on p. 183.

Dehydration fever

This occurs on the third or fourth day in babies who are feeding poorly and have received insufficient fluid. There is usually excessive weight loss (over 10% of birthweight) and a raised serum osmolarity. The babies respond well to rehydration — either oral or intravenous, and the temperature returns to normal.

Cardiac failure

This may be associated with fever at the onset due to an increased metabolic rate (see p. 224).

Intracranial haemorrhage

This may be associated with fever particularly if there is damage to the hypothalamus.

Effects
The effect of fever is to increase fluid losses through the skin, especially if the child is sweating. This leads to hypernatraemia and an increased serum osmolarity. There will also be an increased weight loss. Fever is also associated with increased jaundice and apnoeic episodes.

Management
The cause must be found and treated. Specific treatment of the fever is not usually necessary. However paracetamol can be given, either orally or rectally (12 mg/kg 4–6 hourly up to 4 weeks of age). Sponging the baby with tepid water is also effective; cold water should not be used. The baby should not be placed directly under an electric fan nor by an open window. This simply makes the skin blood vessels vasoconstrict, thus preventing further heat loss so that the baby's core temperature becomes even higher.

HYPOTHERMIA

Causes
Environmental temperature
Babies can become hypothermic if they are in a cold environment or inadequately dressed (see above). If babies need to be nursed naked, either for observation or phototherapy, then appropriate adjustments must be made to the environmental temperature. They may also need to be in an incubator or under a perspex heat shield.

Problems at birth
Babies are particularly susceptible to hypothermia at birth as they are wet so lose heat quickly. Delivery rooms are often not warm enough for the baby and the cot always seems to be placed next to the window. Attention must be paid to these details, especially if the baby is known to be low birthweight. The practice of bathing the newborn in the delivery suite is also guaranteed to cool the babies down. It is unnecessary and is not to be recommended.

Prolonged resuscitation can also contribute to hypothermia unless the baby is dried and warmed properly. Asphyxiated babies have particular difficulties with temperature control anyway.

Babies born at home (unless planned) or on the way to hospital are also susceptible to hypothermia.

Low birthweight babies
Preterm babies and small-for-dates babies are especially liable to develop hypothermia (see p. 124).

Sick babies
Any baby who is very sick may become hypothermic. It is an important sign in septicaemia and other severe infections such as meningitis. Poor peripheral circulation often makes the hands and feet particularly cold.

Hypothermia is also associated with hypoxia, hypoglycaemia and injury to the brain. Babies undergoing an exchange transfusion are prone to hypothermia due to the transfusion of large amounts of cold blood.

Effects
A baby who is simply chilled may have bluish mottling of the skin with a marble pattern (cutis marmorata) on the trunk and limbs. It is due to dilatation of the capillaries and venules and disappears once the baby is warm. It is only seen in the first months of life.

Hypothermia is extremely harmful to babies, especially if they are already sick and it increases their mortality rate. It exacerbates hypoxia and acidosis by increasing oxygen requirement. Respiratory distress is worsened as hypoglycaemia affects surfactant synthesis. It also causes hypoglycaemia. Cold babies are also prone to apnoeic episodes and bradycardia.

Management
As with fever, the prime task is to find and treat the cause. In addition, the baby should be warmed slowly, by 0.5°C/hour. This is best done in an incubator as its environmental temperature

can be accurately controlled. The baby should be wrapped properly and hats are particularly useful. Heat shields may be used and warm water can be put in the incubator's humidifier to create a 'sauna-like' atmosphere.

17: Infection

INTRODUCTION

All newborn babies are susceptible to infection but especially if they are preterm (see p. 122). The immune system is not yet fully mature although transplacentally-acquired antibodies will be of some help in combating certain infections.

It is important that cross-infection is prevented while the baby is in hospital. Medical and nursing personnel must wash their hands using a liquid soap dispenser, and take particular care to dry them thoroughly before touching any baby. Otherwise they can pass on organisms from other babies as well as their own hospital-acquired organisms. Clearly the mother does not need to take these precautions unless she picks up someone else's baby. Staff and visitors with overt infections should keep away from the postnatal ward.

NON-SPECIFIC SIGNS

In some cases the site of infection is obvious, for example in conjunctivitis or umbilical sepsis. However, often the baby is non-specifically unwell and the cause is not readily apparent. This is often the case with the more serious and systemic infections such as septicaemia or meningitis. Non-specific symptoms and signs of infection in a baby include:
- poor feeding;
- persistent vomiting;
- lethargy and excessive sleepiness;
- excessive crying or an abnormally quiet baby;
- apnoeic episode in a preterm baby;

- poor urine output;
- floppiness;
- irritability;
- tachypnoea (respiratory rate > 60/minute);
- cold mottled extremities;
- hypothermia or fever;
- hypoglycaemia;
- jaundice.

More specific signs are discussed with the individual infections.

There may be pointers in the history that suggest the baby has an infection. For example:
- maternal pyrexia during labour;
- prolonged rupture of membranes (see p. 38);
- mother has current infection;
- contact with infection on the ward or from a visitor.

SEPTIC SCREEN

If there is any suggestion that a baby may have an infection then early intervention is necessary. After taking the history, and performing a thorough examination, a full septic screen must be carried out which involves the following steps.

Full blood count with white cell differential. The baby may be anaemic; the normal haemoglobin level is 15–18 g/dl in the newborn. It is also normal to find up to $0.5 \times 10^9/l$ nucleated red cells in peripheral blood in the first 48 hours.

The white count may not be very helpful. The normal total white cell count (WCC) is up to $30 \times 10^9/l$ in the first 48 hours. During this period there are usually more neutrophil polymorphs than lymphocytes but after 48 hours the lymphocytes comprise about 60% of the total WCC. The total WCC given by the Coulter counter is often artificially elevated due to the presence of large nucleated red cells hence the need for a manual differential count. Infection may be associated with a lymphocytic or neutrophil leucocytosis but often the WCC is normal. However after the second day, a neutrophil count $>10 \times 10^9/l$ suggests infection.

Infection may cause a low platelet count (thrombocytopenia)

although sometimes the count is raised as a non-specific response to inflammation. The normal platelet count is 100–300 x 10^9/l in the first week.

Blood culture from a peripheral vein. The skin must be cleaned properly with Betadine otherwise skin commensals (e.g. *Staphylococcus epidermidis*) will contaminate the culture. A minimum of 0.5 ml blood is necessary, although the more blood obtained, the greater the chance of growing the organism. See p. 253 for the techniques of taking blood cultures.

Swabs are taken from the following sites: umbilicus, ear, throat and rectum. Skin swabs should also be taken from any suspicious areas.

Gastric aspirate should be sent in the first few hours of life but only if the baby has not yet been given any milk (see p. 38).

Urine microscopy and culture. A clean-catch urine or suprapubic aspirate is performed (see p. 262). An abnormal microscopy result is signified by >100 white cells per millilitre and the presence of organisms on Gram-staining. A positive culture is a pure growth of >10^5 organisms per millilitre.

Lumbar puncture (LP). There should be a low threshold for performing an LP, particularly after the first 24 hours of life. The technique is described on p. 259. Normal cerebrospinal fluid (CSF) in a neonate should be clear and colourless and contain up to 30 white cells per millilitre, which are predominantly polymorphs. Infection is indicated by cloudy CSF with a raised white count and there will be organisms seen on Gram-staining. If it was a blood-stained tap there will be many white cells in the CSF that have come from the blood. As long as there is less than 1 white cell for every 500 red cells seen, then the extra white cells can be assumed to be from the contaminating blood rather than from infection.

   CSF protein is normally 0.1–2.0 g/l although may be up to 3.0 g/l in preterm babies. It is raised in bacterial infection.

CSF glucose ranges from 2 to 4 mmol/l and is usually about 80% of the blood glucose level. Assuming the baby is not hypoglycaemic, if the CSF glucose is <1 mmol/l or less than 80% of the blood glucose, bacterial infection is indicated.

Chest X-Ray. If the baby is very sick, this should be done on the ward rather than in the X-ray department.

Others. In addition, latex antigen tests or countercurrent immunoelectrophoresis may indicate the presence of certain organisms, namely *Pneumococcus, Meningococcus, Haemophilus influenzae* and *Escherichia coli.* A negative test does not exclude the organism but if positive it is good evidence for the causative organism. The tests can be done on 1.5 ml of clotted blood or on CSF but are not available in every hospital.

The following should also be checked in a sick baby:
• serum sodium, potassium, creatinine and calcium;
• blood glucose (done at the same time as an LP);
• arterial pH, oxygen, carbon dioxide and base excess.

INITIAL TREATMENT

If the baby is very sick, you can not wait for all the microbiology results before starting treatment. An IV cannula is inserted (this can be done at the same time as taking the blood samples) and maintenance fluids given. The child should not be given any oral feeds.

Intravenous antibiotics should be started immediately. Every paediatric department will have their own regime for treating neonatal infection empirically, but here are some suggestions:
• benzylpenicillin plus gentamicin;
• flucloxacillin plus gentamicin;
• ampicillin plus gentamicin;
• cefotaxime (or another third generation cephalosporin) plus benzylpenicillin.
Whenever gentamicin is used, blood levels must be checked before the third dose as high blood levels are associated with deafness and renal toxicity. Trough levels are taken before the

dose is given (should be <2 mg/l) and peak levels 20–30 minutes after the IV dose (should be 6–10 mg/l). 0.5 ml clotted blood is needed.

Once full culture results and antibiotic sensitivities are known, the antibiotics may be adjusted accordingly.

Attention must be paid to the fluid and electrolyte balance, as well as any acidosis or hypotension that often accompanies severe infection.

SPECIFIC INFECTIONS

Specific infections will now be considered with the following format:
- causative organisms;
- clinical presentation;
- investigations;
- treatment;
- sequelae.

Septicaemia

Causative organisms. In neonates, septicaemia accompanies virtually all major infections such as meningitis or pneumonia. The likeliest organisms are group B *Streptococcus*, *Staphylococcus* or *Eschericia coli*.

Clinical presentation. Usually non-specific as outlined above. The baby rapidly becomes very ill.

Investigations. Full septic screen.

Treatment. IV antibiotics for 10–14 days. Start with a cocktail such as benzylpencillin (60 mg/kg/dose 12 hourly if <7 days old or 8 hourly if >7 days old) and gentamicin (2.5 mg/kg/dose 12 hourly if <7 days old or 8 hourly if >7 days old).

If listeriosis is a possibility (see p. 17) then ampicillin should be used instead of benzylpenicillin. Antibiotics may need to be changed once culture results are known.

Sequelae. Sequelae are only likely if the baby suffers bouts of hypotension or hypoxia which may lead to neurological and developmental problems.

Meningitis

Causative organisms. *Escherichia coli* is the most likely organism in this age group, followed by group B *Streptococcus* and *Listeria monocytogenes.* Other possibilities are *Staphylococcus aureus, Meningococcus, Streptococcus faecalis, Haemophilus influenzae* and *Pseudomonas.*

Clinical presentation. Early symptoms are ill-defined and similar to those found in septicaemia. Late features are vomiting, a high-pitched cry, head retraction with an arched back, a bulging anterior fontanelle and convulsions. Hopefully the ill baby will have been noticed before the advent of these late signs. Neck stiffness is rarely seen and photophobia is not detectable in babies.

Investigations. Lumbar puncture is usually diagnostic but sometimes the baby is too unwell for this to be performed. Repeat LPs may be necessary to monitor progress. Blood culture and throat swabs may reveal the organism. Serial head circumference measurements and cranial ultrasound examinations are useful to monitor any enlargement of the ventricles.

Treatment. This depends on the causative organism. There are several possible regimes but our initial IV treatment is ampicillin (50 mg/kg/dose 12 hourly if <7 days old or 8 hourly if >7 days old) and ceftazidime (30 mg/kg/dose 12 hourly).

Treatment is normally for at least 14 days. Other antibiotics that may be helpful are benzylpenicillin, gentamicin and chloramphenicol. Fits should be treated with anticonvulsants (see p. 245).

The babies should be restricted to a fluid intake of 60 ml/kg/day for the first few days as meningitis often causes inappropriate ADH secretion resulting in fluid overload.

Sequelae. There is a 10–20% mortality which is usually due to late diagnosis. 10–30% of the survivors have serious neurological impairment, including obstructive hydrocephalus, deafness, cerebral palsy and mental retardation.

Pneumonia

Causative organisms. Group B *Streptococcus* (particularly if onset is within the first 24 hours) and *Escherichia coli* are the most common. Other possibilities are *Staphylococcus, Pneumococcus, Listeria monocytogenes, Klebsiella* and *Pseudomonas.* Infection with *Mycoplasma* or *Chlamydia* may need to be considered if there is failure to respond to the antibiotics used routinely for pneumonia in the unit. Viral pneumonia is uncommon in the newborn although occasionally outbreaks of respiratory syncytial virus occur.

Clinical presentation. Pneumonia is usually accompanied by septicaemia and the baby has the non-specific symptoms discussed previously. In addition, there may be signs of respiratory distress such as tachypnoea, subcostal recession, and grunting (see p. 206). There may be focal signs on auscultation of the chest (e.g. crepitations) but these do not differentiate pneumonia from other causes of respiratory distress.

Investigations. Blood culture and culture the respiratory secretions. Chest X-ray is usually unhelpful at first, revealing only non-specific changes. Later there may be an area of consolidation (a white patch) or collapse. Occasionally air or fluid-filled spaces (pneumatocoeles) are seen which indicate staphylococcal infection. Arterial blood gases may show a respiratory acidosis with a degree of hypoxaemia.

Treatment. IV antibiotics for 7–10 days. Early onset pneumonia is best treated with benzylpenicillin and gentamicin. After 48 hours of age, *Staphylococcus* is more likely than group B *Streptococcus* so flucloxacillin should replace the benzylpenicillin.

Sequelae. Pneumothorax or empyema are occasionally seen. Late sequelae are rarely seen.

Group B streptococcal infection

Causative organism. Group B β-haemolytic *Streptococcus* (GBS) is the most common organism to cause serious infection in the newborn. It may be acquired *in utero* or at birth from the mother, or alternatively from other sources in late onset disease.

Asymptomatic carriage of GBS in the mother's genital tract is common, and was found in up to 40% of women in some studies. However routine microbiological screening is no longer performed on pregnant women so carriage usually goes undetected.

Clinical presentation. This depends on when the organism is acquired. There tend to be three patterns of infection:

1 *Immediate infection.* The baby may be born with a low Apgar score and need active resuscitation. Usually the babies develop respiratory distress within a few hours of birth. They become tachypnoeic with recession and grunting, rapidly becoming extremely ill. If not treated soon, a fulminant septicaemia develops with a high mortality rate.

2 *Early onset.* Presentation is within 24 hours of birth and is similar to immediate infection. In addition to signs of septicaemia and pneumonia, the babies may develop meningitis.

3 *Late onset.* The babies develop a more insidious infection towards the end of the first week. The majority have meningitis with accompanying septicaemia.

Investigations. Full septic screen is usually necessary. Latex antigen tests may be helpful.

Treatment. IV benzylpenicillin for 10 days. IV gentamicin is also often given as it has synergistic effect with the penicillin. Severe cases may need to be ventilated.

The mainstay of treatment is to start early so rapid recognition of GBS is essential. Every baby who develops overt signs of respiratory distress within 24 hours has GBS until proved otherwise, even if there are other possible explanations for the respiratory difficulties such as hyaline membrane disease in a premature baby. We advocate that all babies on the postnatal ward should have their respiratory rate measured 2 hourly for the first 24 hours. A portable respiratory rate monitor (Graseby MR10) is most suitable as neither the baby nor mother is disturbed during the measurement. If they are tachypnoeic with a rate > 60/minute for two successive readings (the second one should be done 1 hour after the first abnormal reading), the paediatrician must be informed and the baby transferred to the neonatal unit. Assuming the baby was not crying and the tachypnoea is genuine, after 4 hours, the baby is assumed to have GBS until culture results prove otherwise. The baby should have a septic screen and receive IV benzylpenicillin and gentamicin. If blood cultures are negative after 48 hours then the antibiotics may be stopped. Occasionally the baby is still tachypnoeic, and other causes must be excluded (Chapter 19). Although some babies will have received antibiotics unnecessarily, fulminant GBS septicaemia will be prevented by this policy.

Prevention. If the mother is known to be an asymptomatic carrier of GBS the question sometimes arises over prophylaxis for the baby. Some authorities recommend a single dose of intramuscular long-acting penicillin (e.g. one-quarter vial of Triplopen) given after birth. However we do not recommend prophylaxis as there is no evidence that it is any more effective than our policy of careful monitoring for the first 24 hours. There is also no point in giving the mother ampicillin routinely during labour if she is asymptomatic. However if she is pyrexial or there is prolonged rupture of membranes, the mother should receive IV ampicillin and the baby should be screened (see p. 38).

Sequelae. There are none if treatment is initiated in time.

Gastroenteritis
Causative organisms. Usually viral, in particular rotavirus. Bacteria are not often isolated but *Salmonella, Shigella* and enteropathogenic *E. coli* may be the cause.

Clinical presentation. Diarrhoea, which may be preceded by vomiting for up to 48 hours. Gastroenteritis is rare in breastfed babies and is now uncommon in the newborn period.

Investigations. Stool culture or rectal swab for bacteria and viruses. Rotavirus can be detected quickly by electron microscopy or a latex particle agglutination test. Serum electrolytes should be performed if the baby is clinically dehydrated. Daily weights on the same set of weighing scales give the best guide to the state of hydration.

Treatment. Breastfed babies should continue with breast milk but may need additional oral fluids. Bottle-fed babies should stop having milk and be given an oral glucose electrolyte solution such as Dextrolyte or Dioralyte. After 24–48 hours, if the diarrhoea has settled formula milk can be restarted. The baby is gradually regraded to full milk feeds. Initially, milk diluted with water to a quarter-strength is given. If this is tolerated, it is increased every 24 hours, first to half-strength and then three-quarter strength before full milk is given.

Glucose electrolyte solutions should not be given on their own for longer than 48 hours as the baby then develops watery green 'starvation' stools which are difficult to differentiate from the gastroenteritis stools.

Occasionally IV fluids are necessary, but only if the baby is not tolerating anything orally and is losing large amounts of fluid in the stools or vomit. It is safer and easier to rehydrate babies with oral solutions if at all possible.

There is no place for antibiotic treatment unless a specific bacterial organism such as *Salmonella typhi* has been isolated and the baby is systemically unwell.

The baby should be isolated with his mother in a cubicle. Scrupulous hand-washing by medical and nursing staff is essential to prevent an outbreak of gastroenteritis.

Sequelae. Occasionally when milk feeds are reintroduced, the diarrhoea restarts. The baby may have developed a secondary lactose intolerance following the infection. Stool fluid should be tested with a Clinitest tablet soon after it is passed. This diagnosis is likely if the fluid contains more than 0.5% reducing sugars. The baby should be given a lactose-free milk for 6 weeks, and occasionally this is necessary for 2–3 months. Primary lactose tolerance is an extremely rare autosomal recessive condition.

Necrotizing enterocolitis
See Chapter 13, p. 151.

Urinary tract infection (UTI)
Casuative organisms. Escherichia coli is the commonest organism. Other bacteria sometimes grown are *Streptococcus faecalis, Klebsiella, Staphylococcus* and *Pseudomonas.*

Clinical presentation. There are usually only non-specific symptoms hence the need for urine culture whenever a baby is unwell. Any infant with a temperature above 38.5°C with no definite cause must have a urine culture performed. In particular UTI may be associated with persistent vomiting and prolonged jaundice. Delayed diagnosis may lead to septicaemia. If there is pyelonephritis, there may be loin tenderness but this is hard to elicit in a baby. There may also be enlarged kidneys.

Sometimes a urinary tract infection accompanies abnormalities of the genital tract as well as renal and bladder anomalies so the baby must be examined carefully. Posterior urethral valves must be excluded in boys (see p. 109).

Investigations. Urine microscopy and culture are diagnostic (see above). It is essential that a non-contaminated sample of urine is collected. The method we prefer is a clean-catch urine (CCU) as this reduces the rate of contamination from the skin and anus that is so common in urine collected by the bag method. Whilst a negative result from a bag urine is reliable, if it is positive it will have to be confirmed by a clean-catch specimen. This wastes time so it is better to start with a clean-catch urine. If there is any doubt or the baby is septicaemic, the quickest and most reliable method is to perform a suprapubic aspirate (SPA), preferably under ultrasound control. (See p. 262 for details on how to collect urine.) If any organisms are seen on microscopy of SPA urine then a urinary tract infection is confirmed, no matter how many white cells are seen.

If the baby is unwell, blood should be taken for culture as well as serum electrolytes.

Imaging of the renal tract is essential in all children who have a proven urinary tract infection. During the acute illness, the baby should have an ultrasound examination of the kidneys and bladder. A plain abdominal X-ray should also be done to exclude renal stones (very rare in a baby) and abnormalities of the lumbosacral spine. When the infection is treated, a micturating cystourethrogram (MCU) is performed to exclude vesico-ureteric reflux. In addition, a renal isotope scan (e.g. DMSA scan) is carried out 3 months after the infection to detect renal scarring.

Treatment. If the baby is otherwise well, oral antibiotics can be given. Start with trimethoprim (4 mg/kg twice a day) and change only if indicated by culture results. It should be given for 10 days and then the urine is recultured. If the baby is systemically unwell, then IV gentamicin is the drug of choice. Once treatment has finished, antibiotic prophylaxis must be given until the results of the renal imaging are known. This is best done with oral trimethoprim (1–2 mg/kg at night) unless the original infection was resistant to trimethoprim or the baby is not tolerating the drug.

Sequelae. Urinary tract infection is associated with renal scarring and reflux nephropathy. Without proper long-term management, this is associated with hypertension and chronic renal failure in later life.

Umbilical sepsis
Causative organisms. Staphylococcus aureus or *Escherichia coli.*

Clinical presentation. The stump from the umbilical cord normally separates from the umbilicus after about 7 days. During the first few days, the area is often moist and sometimes it appears to be sticky as if covered in pus. This does not necessarily mean the stump is infected although when moist it can certainly act as a good medium for bacterial growth. However if the skin around the separating cord appears red, and especially if it is also hot and shiny, a local cellulitis is present. This is potentially very serious as the infection can spread via the remnant of the umbilical vessels to the liver and cause a dangerous portal pyaemia.

Investigations. Superficial skin swab and if the baby appears unwell blood cultures should also be taken.

Treatment. A 'sticky' cord needs to be kept clean. It should be washed regularly with sterile saline or surgical spirit, and antiseptic powder is applied when the surgical spirit has evaporated. Alcohol inactivates hexachlorophane which is the antiseptic commonly used in powders.

If a red flare is present in the surrounding skin, antibiotics are necessary. If it is minor, oral flucloxacillin (25 mg/kg/dose 6 hourly for 5 days) is sufficient. If however it is a large area or the baby has any non-specific signs of systemic infection at all, IV flucloxacillin (same dose as oral) and gentamicin should be given for 7 days.

Sequelae. Chronic low grade infection can lead to formation of an umbilical granuloma (see p. 95).

Skin pustules
Causative organisms. Staphylococcus aureus.

Clinical presentation. Clusters of yellow pustules which first appear on the fourth day or later are usually due to infection. They tend to be in the axilla or groin but can appear anywhere on the skin. They are often difficult to differentiate from toxic erythema (see p. 202) although the latter tend to appear earlier. If there is any doubt, the spots should be assumed to be staphylococcal pustules.

Investigations. Prick the pustule with a sterile fine needle and send a swab of the contents for culture.

Treatment. Oral flucloxacillin for 5 days unless the baby is unwell in which case the antibiotics should be given intravenously.

Sequelae. None.

Scalded skin syndrome
Causative organisms. An exotoxin-producing *Staphylococcus aureus.*

Clinical presentations. This is also known as toxic epidermal necrolysis. The whole picture can develop within hours or it may take a few days. At first there are tender areas of red skin. Large flaccid blisters appear and then the outer layer of skin peels away leaving raw areas that resemble a scald. It predominantly affects the face, neck, axillae and groins but sometimes the infection is more localized. It may be accompanied by conjunctivitis and the perioral region is often involved although the mucosa is spared. There is marked fluid loss through the raw skin and there is usually a low-grade fever.

Investigations. Superficial skin swab and blood cultures.

Treatment. IV flucloxacillin for 7 days. Intravenous fluids will need to be given at first.

Sequelae. The baby recovers within 5–7 days. There is no residual skin scarring.

Bullous impetigo
Causative organisms. Staphylococcus aureus. Occasionally β-haemolytic streptococci are responsible.

Clinical presentation. This is a bullous or vesicular form of impetigo seen in the newborn. The blisters vary from small vesicles to large flaccid bullae filled with pale yellow fluid. Blisters are especially found in the axillae, groins and on the hands. When they rupture, an area of raw skin is exposed.

Investigations. Superficial skin swab or culture fluid from a bullous. Blood cultures should also be taken.

Treatment. The babies should be barrier-nursed. They are given IV flucloxacillin for 7 days for staphylococci. If streptococci are isolated, IV benzylpenicillin is given for 10 days. The skin should also be cleaned with an antiseptic such as hexachlorophane (Ster-Zac powder), 3–4 times a day until new lesions stop appearing.

Sequelae. None.

Paronychia
Causative organisms. Staphylococcus aureus.

Clinical presentation. There is a reddening of the skin along the side of the nail bed of a finger or toe. It may be swollen and tender and can affect several digits.

Investigations. Superficial skin swab.

Treatment. Oral flucloxacillin for 10 days.

Sequelae. If untreated it can act as a source of *Staphylococcus* which can disseminate and cause systemic or more serious infections.

Breast abscess
Causative organisms. Staphylococcus aureus.

Clinical presentation. Hormonal changes at birth sometimes lead to breast engorgement which in turn can cause acute mastitis. Sometimes this is followed by formation of an abscess. There is a red tender swelling of the breast or sometimes just part of it. It is usually accompanied by axillary lymphadenopathy on the same side. It must be differentiated from simple physiological breast engorgement which can also be unilateral.

Investigations. Superficial skin swab and culture any pus if surgery is required.

Treatment. IV flucloxacillin for 10 days. Incision and drainage may be necessary if there is a localized fluctant area.

Sequelae. None.

Thrush
Causative organisms. The fungus *Candida albicans.*

Clinical presentation. Oral infection produces white plaques on the tongue and inside of the mouth which are surrounded by a red ring of inflamed mucosa. The plaques are firmly attached and can not be scraped off the surface unlike particles of curdled milk which often resemble thrush. The baby may be reluctant to feed.

Thrush also commonly causes a rash around the perineum in the nappy area. It is a bright red rash with discrete satellite lesions (a few spots set apart from the main rash). Spots are also found within the skin creases of the groin which differentiates it from the common nappy rash of ammoniacal dermatitis (see p. 203) in which the skin creases are spared.

Investigations. Superficial skin swab.

Treatment. Oral thrush is treated with miconazole gel (twice a day) which should be continued for 2 days after the lesions have disappeared. The perineal infection is treated with miconazole cream (applied after each nappy change) until the rash has been clear for 1 week. An alternative is to use nystatin suspension (1 ml 6 hourly) in the mouth and nystatin cream on the skin although it is slower acting than miconazole. There is no point in treating the mouth and not the perineum and vice versa as infection is nearly always present in both areas simultaneously.

Sequelae. A breastfed baby can pass on oral thrush to the mother which can colonize cracked nipples (see p. 137).

Conjunctivitis

Causative organisms. It is usually due to *Staphylococcus, Escherichia coli, Streptococcus* or *Haemophilus.* Sometimes it is due to *Chlamydia trachomatis* or *Gonococcus.* Conjunctivitis may also be chemical, for example chlorhexidine used in swabbing the mother's perineum may get in the baby's eyes at delivery. In some countries, silver nitrate drops are instilled in all babies' eyes as prophylaxis against gonococcal conjunctivitis and this may lead to a severe chemical conjunctivitis.

Clinical presentation. Many babies have sticky eyes for the first day or two and this does not necessarily imply there is infection present. This irritation tends to clear spontaneously. However if there is a later presentation or the eye is more than just sticky, then infection should be assumed. There tends to be redness, swelling and a purulent discharge which presents at around 3–5 days and this is usually due to the commoner bacteria mentioned above.

Chlamydia trachomatis usually presents later at around 7 days of age. Suspicion should also be aroused with persistent conjunctivitis that is resistant to standard treatment. There may be a history of maternal STD (sexually transmitted disease) — see p. 23.

Gonococcal conjunctivitis (see also p. 18) causes a profuse purulent discharge and may involved deeper structures of the eye. It classically presents on the first day but may appear any time within the first week. There may be a history of maternal STD.

Investigations. Standard swabs of the discharge will reveal all bacteria but will be sterile in chlamydial infection. Special swabs are necessary for *Chlamydia* and the microbiology department should be contacted in advance. Culturing for *Chlamydia* tends to be done only after conventional treatment has failed, unless there is a positive maternal history. If *Gonococcus* is suspected, urgent Gram-staining of the pus is carried out and will reveal Gram-negative diplococci. Special arrangements for immediate culture of swabs is needed.

Treatment. Sticky eyes need only be cleansed regularly with sterile saline.

Treatment of conjunctivitis should start with neomycin eye ointment four times a day for 5 days. Both eyes should be treated, with separate tubes of ointment for each eye. Ointment is preferable to eye-drops as the antibiotic stays in contact with the eye for a longer period.

If there is no improvement after this time and culture was sterile, the chlamydial swabs are taken and 0.5% chloramphenicol ointment started. If *Chlamydia* is isolated, chlortetracycline ointment (6 hourly) is used for 2 weeks as well as oral erythromycin (30 mg/kg/dose 12 hourly) for 2 weeks. The reason for not starting treatment of all cases of conjunctivitis with chloramphenicol is that the antibiotic will render *Chlamydia* swabs negative. But at the same time chloramphenicol alone will only partially treat the conjunctivitis if *Chlamydia* are present.

Gonococcal conjunctivitis is treated with 0.5% chloramphenicol drops applied half-hourly (drops are given when the antibiotic is used with this frequency), and then 0.5% chloramphenicol ointment applied 2 hourly for 3 days. In addition the infant needs IV benzylpenicillin (25 mg/kg/dose 12 hourly) for 7 days.

Sequelae. Occasionally severe conjunctivitis can lead to infection of the lacrimal sac (dacrocystitis). There is a tender deep red swelling on the medial side of the lower lid. Gentle pressure over the swelling will lead to purulent discharge from the lacrimal duct and this should be performed 3–4 times a day. 0.5% chloramphenicol ointment and IV flucloxacillin are necessary.

In 2% of babies there is a congenital obstruction of the nasolacrimal (tear) duct. This is usually due to delay in canalization of the duct and tends to clear spontaneously. However occasionally it leads to persistent infection and the condition should be considered in cases of recurrent or persistent conjunctivitis or dacrocystitis. The infant should be referred to an ophthalmologist.

Gonococcal infection can occasionally lead to blindness as well as systemic manifestations such as pneumonia, meningitis and arthritis.

Osteomyelitis and septic arthritis
Causative organisms. Staphylococcus aureus usually. Other possibilities include group B *Streptococcus, Haemophilus influenzae* and rarely *Gonococcus.*

Clinical presentation. Particularly in the case of *Staphylococcus*, there may be a pre-existing local source of infection such as a paronychia or other superficial skin infection.

It is very difficult to tell bone and joint infection apart on clinical grounds so they are dealt with together. Often there are no specific signs, just an ill infant who will not feed. Reluctance to move a limb (pseudoparalysis) or crying when the limb is moved or touched are valuable localizing signs. Swelling and redness over the lesion appears late. Common sites for osteomyelitis are the head of the femur, the humerus and the maxilla.

Investigations. Blood cultures may reveal the pathogen. An X-ray of the limb should be taken immediately as soft tissue swelling or a raised and thickened periosteum are seen at an early stage in neonatal osteomyelitis (unlike in older children where the X-ray is normal for the first 10 days). A fractured bone from birth trauma will also be excluded. If the X-ray is normal but the clinical signs indicate that there is a bone or joint problem, an isotope bone scan may be helpful. The scan may show a 'hot spot' over an area of osteomyelitis.

Treatment. IV ampicillin and flucloxacillin are given for at least 3 weeks, followed by at least 3 weeks of oral treatment. Surgical drainage is occasionally necessary.

Sequelae. These mainly result from a missed or delayed diagnosis. The infection may spread to a neighbouring joint from the bone or systemically to the brain or lungs. Chronic osteomyelitis can also follow with a discharging sinus and bone growth can be affected.

Otitis media

Causative organisms. Group B *Streptococcus, Pneumococcus, Haemophilus influenzae* and several viruses.

Clinical presentation. Whilst infection of the middle ear is uncommon in the newborn, the diagnosis is often missed as it is not usually considered. Infants with cleft palate are particularly prone to this infection. The infants have non-specific signs such as irritability, poor feeding and vomiting. The ear drum is hard to visualize in the newborn but if it seen to be bright red or dull it implies infection.

Investigations. Aspiration of the middle ear is diagnostic but rarely justified.

Treatment. Oral ampicillin and flucloxacillin for 7 days.

Sequelae. There are no sequelae in the neonate.

CONGENITAL INFECTIONS

Congenital viral infections and toxoplasmosis have been dealt with in Chapters 2 and 9. Congenital syphilis and listeriosis is also dealt with in Chapter 2.

Chicken pox

Congenital varicella zoster, its prevention and treatment is discussed on p. 20.

The baby can also acquire varicella from contacts such as siblings, hospital staff and other babies on the ward. In addition a non-immune mother may be in contact with the infection. Cases are infective from 1–2 days before the rash appears until the last vesicles have crusted. In all cases, if the mother has never had chicken pox the baby is vulnerable as he will have no passively-acquired antibodies. The baby should receive 0.5 ml ZIG intramuscularly. If the mother is sure that she has had chicken pox in the past then no further action is required.

Infection can be confirmed by electron microscopy of some vesicle fluid obtained by pricking a lesion with a sterile needle.

Treatment is IV acyclovir (10 mg/kg/dose 8 hourly) for 7 days.

FURTHER READING

Report of a Working Group of the Research Unit, Royal College of Physicians. (1991) Guidelines for the management of acute urinary tract infection in childhood. *Journal of the Royal College of Physicians of London* **25**: 36–41.

18: Rashes

Rashes are extremely common in babies and although they may appear alarming to the parents they are usually of no significance. Many of the rashes have a similar appearance but with experience they can usually be differentiated from one another. It is worthwhile looking through one of the many atlases of paediatric dermatology to familiarize yourself with the appearances of the commoner rashes. Common birthmarks (naevi) have been dealt with on p. 98.

TOXIC ERYTHEMA

This rash is extremely common and it is seen in over 50% of fullterm babies, although it is rare in premature babies. It is also known as erythema toxicum or erythema neonatorum. It is seen in the first week of life and tends to appear within the first 48 hours. It varies in severity from a few spots to a blotchy rash that can cover most of the body apart from the palms and soles. The spots tend to be found on the trunk, face and limbs but their distribution fluctuates from day to day. The spots consist of red macules which can be up to 2–3 cm in size, with a central white or pale yellow vesicle. The spots must be differentiated from pustules due to *Staphylococcus* and if there is any doubt a swab should be taken. The contents of the vesicles are sterile but contain eosinophils. The cause is unknown and no treatment is necessary. The rash disappears spontaneously after a few days.

MILIA

These tiny spots are commonly seen on the face, particularly on the forehead, cheeks and around the nose. They are 1–2 mm papules which are usually white but may be yellow. They are retention cysts due to clogging of the sebaceous glands with keratin and sebaceous material. The cysts rupture and disappear within a few weeks. No treatment is necessary.

SEBACEOUS GLAND HYPERPLASIA

The appearance is similar to milia except that the spots may be larger and more abundant. They consist of yellow papules found mainly on the nose, cheeks and around the mouth. They are due to maternal androgen stimulation and disappear after a few weeks. No treatment is necessary.

HEAT RASH

This is also known as miliaria and is due to sweat retention in the sweat glands of a baby that is too warm and humid. The rash consists of red vesicles that can occur anywhere but tend to be found on the face, neck, trunk and skin creases. They disappear once the baby is cooled down and are sometimes present for only a short time.

TRANSIENT NEONATAL PUSTULAR MELANOSIS

This condition is also called transient neonatal pustulosis. The name is slightly misleading as the clear vesicular lesions are sterile and not strictly pustules. It is uncommon and consists of multiple vesicles which can occur anywhere but are most commonly found on the neck and trunk. Unlike toxic erythema the vesicles are not associated with surrounding erythema and are usually present at birth. After a few days the lesions either rupture and disappear or dry out leaving a brown crust which can be gently scraped off the skin. Hyperpigmented macules may persist for up to 3 months.

NAPPY RASHES

In the neonatal period, nappy rashes tend to be due to irritation from faeces and so are mainly perianal. The typical nappy rash which is due to irritation of the skin by urine-soaked nappies is commoner after the first month of life. It is a contact dermatitis (also known as ammoniacal dermatitis) and is initially confined to the skin under the nappy. When severe it also involves the upper thighs and lower abdomen. The skin creases in the groin tend to be spared which differentiates it from thrush which includes the skin creases. The skin is red and inflamed and may even break down. It is sore and makes the baby miserable.

The dermatitis can be avoided by regular nappy changes and it is seen less often with the modern disposable nappies. The rash can be treated with a barrier cream (such as zinc and castor oil) which protects the skin from further irritation and allows it to heal. Exposure to the air is the best way of treating the rash but leaving a baby without a nappy is somewhat messy and inconvenient in the home. Occasionally a steriod-containing cream is indicated if the skin is severely inflamed, and this is best combined with an antifungal preparation as there is often a secondary infection.

The second commonest form of nappy rash is candidiasis. Its presentation and treatment have been discussed on p. 196.

INFANTILE SEBORRHOEIC DERMATITIS

This is may appear in the first weeks of life but is more often seen after 3–4 months. It consists of red scaly skin lesions which are greasy and at first involve the skin creases and the nappy area, particularly around the groin. Later it can affect the scalp, neck, behind the ears and axillae. On the scalp it is known as cradle cap. It does not bother the baby but is rather unsightly. It usually clears up within a few weeks, but it is prone to secondary infection with bacteria or fungi. If treatment is necessary, a cream containing hydrocortisone and an antifungal is used. Cradle cap can be treated with a cream containing sulphur and salicylic acid.

STAPHYLOCOCCAL SKIN INFECTIONS

Skin infections due to *Staphylococcus aureus* can cause pustules, scalded skin syndrome and bullous impetigo. These have been discussed in Chapter 17.

PURPURA

Purpura refers to tiny red or purple spots that are due to capillary haemorrhages in the skin. The spots do not blanche when you press on them. Purpura confined to the head may result from pressure on the neck or face at delivery, or if the cord was tightly round the baby's neck. This is often accompanied by traumatic cyanosis (see p. 71).

When purpura is generalized, it is usually due to a deficiency of platelets, so the baby's platelet count must be checked. This most commonly follows maternal idiopathic thrombocytopenia (see p. 7). Neonatal thrombocytopenia can also result from the mother taking chlorothiazide diuretics during the pregnancy.

In a sick baby, purpura may be due to septicaemia or congenital infections such as rubella, cytomegalovirus or toxoplasmosis.

ACNE NEONATORUM

Infantile acne usually develops after 3 months of age, but it is occasionally seen in younger babies when it is termed acne neonatorum. It is commoner in boys. The acne comprises papules and comedones (plugs of grease in sebaceous glands) and rarely pustules, nodules and cysts. Lesions are found mainly on the cheeks, forehead and chin. The acne tends to resolve by 1–2 years of age but can persist to puberty. It is best to simply clean the face with mild soap and water, avoiding creams and lotions. Special preparations are available for severe cases.

EPIDERMOLYSIS BULLOSA

This is a group of inherited disorders in which blisters and erosions appear on the skin after minor pressure. They vary markedly in severity and some forms are lethal. Referral to a specialist centre is required.

FURTHER READING

Verbov J (1988) *Essential Paediatric Dermatology.* Clinical Press Ltd, Bristol.

19: Breathing Difficulties

CLINICAL FEATURES

When a newborn has difficulty breathing he is said to have respiratory distress. Whatever the cause, the presentation is similar. The usual signs are:
• raised respiratory rate; over 60/minute (tachypnoea);
• grunting — a grunt or squeak heard at the end of expiration;
• subcostal and intercostal recession, sternal retraction;
• nasal flaring.
In addition the baby may be cyanosed.

INITIAL INVESTIGATIONS

Chest X-ray. This may be diagnostic but changes are often non-specific at first. If possible the X-ray should be taken in the X-ray department as better films will be obtained but it may be necessary for a doctor to accompany the infant.

Arterial blood gas. There may be respiratory acidosis with a degree of hypoxia. This is indicated by:
• low pH <7.30;
• low P_{O_2} <9 kPa;
• high P_{CO_2} >6 kPa;
• normal bicarbonate 18–21 mmol/l;
• normal base deficit <5 mmol/l.

Nitrogen washout test. It is occasionally necessary to perform this test on a cyanosed baby to indicate whether the cyanosis is due to pulmonary or cardiac disease. It is described on p. 220.

CAUSES

The causes fall into four categories:
1 Pulmonary.
2 Cardiac.

3 Central nervous system disorders.
4 Neuromuscular.

Pulmonary causes

Hyaline membrane disease
The name derives from the amorphous membranes that line the terminal bronchioles and alveoli in this disease. It is also known as idiopathic respiratory distress syndrome (IRDS) or respiratory distress syndrome (RDS).

Preterm babies are particularly susceptible to this condition and it is the commonest cause of death in babies born before a gestation of 36 weeks. Hyaline membrane disease (HMD) is almost inevitable in babies born before 30 weeks. It is also common in infants of diabetic mothers.

The condition is due to a deficiency of pulmonary surfactant which is poorly produced before the 34th week of gestation. Surfactant is a substance normally present on the alveolar walls which has the effect of lowering the surface tension within the alveolar sacs. Without surfactant, the smaller alveoli tend to collapse at the end of expiration and a pressure greater than the baby is able to generate is required to re-expand them. Meanwhile the larger alveoli are still easily expanded and this leads to uneven ventilation within the lung. Eventually respiratory failure ensues.

Onset of respiratory distress is usually within 3–4 hours although may be sooner in very premature babies. As well as tachypnoea, grunting and recession, the babies develop central cyanosis. There is poor chest expansion with reduced breath sounds and crepitations may be heard.

The chest X-ray will often be normal in the first few hours. Later the lung fields show a fine reticular pattern and may then appear opaque with the classic 'ground-glass' appearance. The contrast between the air in the bronchi and the dense lung fields produces an air bronchogram.

The babies need to be nursed on a neonatal unit. Mild cases may only need to be given oxygen in a headbox. Most cases however, require ventilatory support with regular arterial blood gas monitoring. Artificial surfactant has recently been developed and is given by instillation down the endotracheal tube in infants with severe disease, sometimes with dramatic effects. The babies should not be fed but be given IV fluids. Intravenous antibiotics are necessary as respiratory distress syndrome can not be differentiated from group B streptococcal pneumonia until blood culture results are known. In addition, preterm babies are susceptible to infection and it is possible that a baby with hyaline membrane disease also has pneumonia.

Depending on the degree of prematurity, most cases begin to improve within a week. This is indicated by a decrease in ventilatory requirement. Unfortunately some babies will develop chronic lung disease with a long-term oxygen requirement.

Pneumonia

Pneumonia, particularly when due to group B *Streptococcus* can cause early onset respiratory distress. The subject is dealt with on p. 188.

Pneumonia can also follow aspiration of milk. This is commoner in premature babies as they have a poor cough reflex and are also prone to gastro-oesophageal reflux. This means that material such as regurgitated milk in the pharynx is easily aspirated into the lungs. Babies with poorly coordinated swallowing due to neurological problems are also at risk. Signs may be minimal and are often limited to mild tachypnoea but a chest X-ray may show extensive changes, usually in the right upper lobe. IV antibiotics and physiotherapy are required.

Rarely, a tracheo-oesophageal fistula produces no gross symptoms during the first feed, especially when there is no accompanying oesophageal atresia. The infant may then present with pneumonia due to milk passing through the fistula. Usually, however, babies with this anomaly have choking and coughing spasms at the start of each feed.

Transient tachypnoea of the newborn (TTN)

Raised respiratory rate and grunting from birth or within 3 hours is sometimes found in fullterm infants and resolves within 48 hours. The chest X-ray often shows a streaky appearance in the lung fields with fluid in the fissures but may be normal. The syndrome may be due to failure of reabsorption of lung fluids at birth or a mild form of respiratory distress syndrome. Oxygen given into a headbox may be needed. Intravenous antibiotics must be given until blood culture results are known as the syndrome can not be differentiated from group B streptococcal pneumonia in the early stages.

Pneumothorax

Pneumothorax is the presence of air within the pleural cavity which may lead to collapse of the lung on the same side. It results from overinflation and rupture of alveoli so can follow intermittent positive pressure ventilation given whilst resuscitating an asphyxiated baby. It may also occur as a result of vigorous spontaneous respiratory efforts of such a baby, particularly if the baby is making an effort to overcome an airways obstruction (e.g. from a plug of mucus or meconium). Pneumothoraces most commonly occur during ventilation of premature babies and are the result of high ventilatory pressures and underlying lung disease. A common cause is displacement of the endotracheal tube into the right main bronchus which means all the ventilatory pressure is confined to one lung.

The clinical picture tends to fall into three patterns:

1 Rapid deterioration and sudden collapse of the baby. This results from a tension pneumothorax which leads to displacement of the mediastinum to the opposite side and compression of the heart, as well as collapse of the lung on the affected side. This diagnosis must be considered in any infant who deteriorates rapidly for no obvious reason. There is no time for an X-ray. This is a life-threatening emergency and its management is dealt with on p. 55.

2 There may be a more gradual onset of respiratory distress. Symptoms of dyspnoea may be accompanied by hyper-resonance and reduced breath sounds on the affected side, and the chest may be asymmetrical. Diagnosis can be confirmed by a chest X-ray, the absence of normal lung markings being the most important sign. A chest drain connected to an underwater seal will need to be inserted into the pleural cavity to remove the air and re-expand the lung.

3 The pneumothorax may be asymptomatic and an incidental

finding on a chest X-ray. X-ray surveys have shown an incidence of approximately 1% of spontaneous asymptomatic pneumothoraces in the newborn. No treatment is necessary as the small amount of air in the pleural cavity is slowly absorbed.

Meconium aspiration
When a fullterm fetus is distressed before delivery meconium may be passed and there is a risk of this being aspirated into the lungs. Management of meconium deliveries is described on p. 68. Unfortunately some of these babies start respiratory movements before there has been an opportunity to clear the mouth and pharynx of meconium and aspiration is then inevitable.

Inhaled meconium may cause bronchial obstruction and air-trapping, so there is a high risk of developing a pneumothorax or pneumomediastinum as the infant breathes against an obstruction. Airway obstruction may also lead to secondary collapse and subsequent infection of the distal segments of the lungs. There is mismatched ventilation and perfusion of the lungs and right-to-left shunting of blood through the lungs leads to marked hypoxia. The babies need mechanical ventilation and antibiotics are mandatory. The babies are usually very sick and recovery takes about 7–10 days.

Congenital causes
There are some rare causes of respiratory distress due to congenital anomalies that affect the respiratory tract.
1 *Pulmonary hypoplasia* is often the result of oligohydramnios and may be associated with Potter's syndrome (see p. 109). There is a narrow chest and it is extremely difficult to ventilate the baby. The condition is usually fatal, particularly in premature babies.
2 *Diaphragmatic hernia* may present with difficulty in resuscitating the baby (see p. 56). Alternatively there may be tachypnoea with vomiting and a flat appearance to the abdomen. There may be a normal or impaired percussion note over the chest wall. The breath sounds are normal or decreased whilst bowel sounds may be heard in the chest. Since a diaphragmatic hernia is most commonly left-sided, the heart is usually displaced over to the right so the diagnosis should be suspected in apparent dextrocar-

dia. Chest X-ray may show loops of small intestine or solid organs in the thorax. However it may take 12 hours from birth for air to reach the colon and produce the characteristic appearance. A large nasogastric tube is necessary to keep the stomach empty and intubation may be necessary. It is sometimes difficult to ventilate the baby as the lung is usually hypoplastic on the affected side. Transfer to a neonatal surgical unit is mandatory.

3 *Congenital lobar emphysema* may present at any time but is seen most commonly in the neonatal period. It is caused by gross overdistension of one lobe, usually the left upper lobe. The overinflated lobe causes herniation of the lung across the midline and depression of the diaphragm. The heart and entire mediastinum may be pushed across to the opposite side which may cause compression collapse of the other lung.

Lobar emphysema may result from an abnormality of the cartilaginous rings surrounding one of the major bronchi to a lobe. The unsupported bronchial walls collapse and cause a 'check valve' obstruction: with powerful inspiratory efforts air is forced past the obstruction but cannot be expelled, so the lobe becomes greatly overexpanded. There is also deficient elastic tissue so the affected lobe cannot deflate normally.

There is increasing respiratory distress with a very high respiratory rate and often central cyanosis. The chest X-ray can be difficult to interpret. The affected side will be translucent and if the mediastinum is displaced the diagnosis must be differentiated from a tension pneumothorax. If the affected lobe clearly shows lung markings then a pneumothorax is excluded. Mild cases improve spontaneously but if there is severe dyspnoea an emergency thoracotomy and lobectomy are required.

4 *Cystic adenomatoid malformation* of the lung is due to excessive overgrowth of terminal bronchiolar structures which tends to affect the lower lobes. Most cases present in the newborn with varying degrees of respiratory distress, often within hours of birth. Chest X-ray shows an opaque lung field with irregular cystic areas. A congenital diaphragmatic hernia has a similar appearance on X-ray so a nasogastric tube must be inserted to identify the position of the stomach. The abdomen should also be included in the X-ray to look for a normal gas pattern. With aeration the cysts continue to expand and may compress the rest of the lung and lead to mediastinal shift. Ventilation is sometimes needed and urgent surgical referral is necessary for a lobectomy.

5 *Congenital laryngeal stridor* is also known as laryngomalacia. It causes persistent inspiratory stridor in infancy and is frequently present from birth. When the baby is breathing quietly, it may be hardly noticeable but can be quite marked if the baby cries or has a cold. There may occasionally be mild respiratory distress with recession. If the child is feeding well and not distressed, intervention is not required. It is worthwhile checking an arterial or capillary blood gas to ensure CO_2 is not being retained. Symptoms lessen as the laryngeal tissues become firmer and chest wall compliance improves. Most children grow out of the problem by 1–2 years.

6 *Choanal atresia or stenosis.* Congenital obstruction to air passing through the nose causes the newborn considerable difficulty as he depends upon a clear nasal airway. Choanal atresia is a posterior nasal obstruction and when bilateral can present with respiratory distress (see p. 104).

7 *Pierre Robin syndrome* may lead to respiratory distress if the tongue falls backwards and occludes the airway (see p. 104).

Congenital heart disease

Dyspnoea during feeding, reluctance to feed and a rapid respiratory rate with recession may indicate heart failure. Excessive weight gain and enlargement of the liver are early confirmatory signs. Cardiac failure is dealt with on p. 224.

Central nervous system

Disorders of the central nervous system (CNS) may cause apnoea, slow gasping respirations or periodic breathing.

Drugs

Narcotic analgesia such as pethidine given to the mother before delivery may cause apnoea in the newborn. The baby may need to be intubated and should receive a narcotic antagonist such as naloxone (see p. 67).

Cerebral birth trauma

This may inhibit the onset of spontaneous respiratory movements after birth so that it is necessary to intubate and ventilate the baby.

Often however, there are no symptoms until 48 hours after delivery when an apnoeic episode occurs. Apnoea is defined as cessation of respiration for more than 10 seconds. It may lead to hypoxia, cyanosis and bradycardia and usually the baby starts to breathe again spontaneously. When respiratory movements recommence, they are often slow and gasping or have a pattern of increasing and decreasing depth which is known as periodic breathing.

These symptoms are due to raised intracranial pressure, but are non-specific. Many normal premature babies have bouts of irregular respiratory movements and periodic breathing. In addition similar clinical features may be seen with hypoxaemia, hypoglycaemia, meningitis and intraventricular haemorrhage.

Apnoea of prematurity

Recurrent apnoeic episodes are common in premature babies of less than 32 weeks gestation. The babies are otherwise perfectly well and the apnoeas usually begin when the babies are a few days old. The apnoea may be accompanied by bradycardia and a fall in oxygen saturation. Despite much research the cause is still not certain but is probably of central origin.

The diagnosis can only be made once all other causes of apnoeic episodes are excluded as an apnoea may be the first non-specific sign of many serious conditions. These include:
• pulmonary disease (e.g. respiratory distress syndrome, pneumothorax),
• airway obstruction or aspiration of feed;
• septicaemia and other major infections;
• hypoglycaemia;
• hypocalcaemia;
• intracranial haemorrhage;
• convulsions (which may be misdiagnosed as an apnoea);
• cardiac failure (especially with pulmonary oedema).

An apnoeic episode can usually be curtailed by gently stimulating the baby or flicking his feet. All premature babies should be connected to an apnoea monitor, usually until they are old enough to go into a cot. Recurrent episodes may require treatment with intravenous aminophylline or oral theophylline. It is important to monitor blood theophylline levels. Occasionally ventilatory support is necessary.

Neuromuscular
Occasionally a neuromuscular disorder is severe enough to affect the respiratory muscles.

Congenital myotonic dystrophy
One of the commonest muscle diseases to present in the newborn is congenital myotonic dystrophy. It is a dominantly inherited disorder, usually passed on by the mother who is only mildly affected or not even diagnosed. Diagnosis in the mother should be suspected if she has difficulty releasing her grip when you shake her hand. The incidence is one in 3500 live births. Mildly affected babies are hypotonic and may have difficulty sucking and swallowing so that there may have been polyhydramnios. When severe, the babies are asphyxiated at birth and require ventilation due to poor respiratory effort. The face has a characteristic appearance with a triangular shaped mouth and facial diplegia. There may also be limb contractures. If the baby requires ventilation for more than 4 weeks survival is unlikely.

Myasthenia gravis
Babies of mothers with myasthenia gravis may have respiratory problems if severely affected (see p. 8).

Spinal muscular atrophy
This autosomal recessive disorder is also known as Werdnig-Hoffmann disease. It is a lower motor neurone disease with variable manifestations. The babies are hypotonic and may have severe limb weakness or even paralysis. The facial muscles however are spared so that the baby appears alert. When severe, the respiratory muscles are also affected which leads to progressive respiratory difficulties.

Miscellaneous

Severe anaemia

The acute onset of severe anaemia will lead to tachypnoea. This may be due to acute haemorrhage at birth and management is described on p. 56.

Metabolic acidaemia

This may lead to tachypnoea due to acid–base homeostatic mechanisms. Causes include hypoxia, hypotension, sepsis, anaemia and inborn errors of metabolism.

Snuffly babies

In the first weeks of life, excessive nasal secretions that block the nose are common. It is usually a clear mucoid discharge and rarely is it due to infection. However it can interfere with feeding and cause parental anxiety. If there are feeding problems, 0.9% sodium chloride nose drops can be used before feeds but it is better to give the parents a mucus extractor and teach them to gently suck out the baby's nose before the feed starts.

FURTHER READING

Dinwiddie R (1990) *The Diagnosis and Management of Paediatric Respiratory Disease.* Churchill Livingstone, Edinburgh.

20: Heart Problems

Congenital heart disease refers to structural or functional heart disease that is present at birth, even if it is not diagnosed until much later. It is common with an incidence of eight per 1000 live births. Three of these eight will have disease severe enough to be life-threatening. These figures exclude rates for bicuspid aortic valves which affect 2% of the population, and patent ductus arteriosus in premature babies which is often transient and so common as to almost be considered normal. There is an even higher incidence of cardiac defects in stillbirths and spontaneous abortions.

The high incidence of structural defects is hardly surprising when you consider the embryological formation of the heart. It begins as a hollow tube and ends as a complex four-chambered structure with valves and multiple vascular connections. In general, structural defects consist of holes, blockages or misconnections. Sometimes several lesions coexist which results in complex heart disease.

It is likely that congenital heart disease arises from a combination of genetic susceptibility and environmental insult. The genetic abnormality may occur on any one of a number of genes responsible for formation of the heart. However the genetic abnormality must combine with an environmental factor that occurs during the embryonic stage of cardiac development, which is between the second and ninth week of pregnancy. Monozygotic twins have double the incidence of heart defects.

Certain inherited disorders are frequently associated with heart disease. For example in Marfan's syndrome, most patients have evidence of aortic dilatation or mitral valve prolapse. In Noonan's syndrome, half the patients have a heart defect, usually involving the pulmonary valve.

Up to 10% of infants with a heart lesion have a detectable chromosomal abnormality. 40% of babies with Down's syndrome have congenital heart disease, most commonly an atrioventricular canal defect. 20% of babies with Turner's syndrome have coarctation of the aorta or aortic stenosis. The incidence of congenital heart disease in Trisomy 13 (Patau's syndrome), and Trisomy 18 (Edward's syndrome) is 80–90%.

There are a number of environmental factors that have been identified as contributing to the aetiology of congenital heart disease. Certain drugs taken in pregnancy are implicated, including alcohol, amphetamines, phenytoin, lithium, oestrogens and progestogens. Congenital viral infections, particularly rubella, may affect the heart. Maternal diabetes mellitus has a 5% risk of a structural heart defect in the fetus, particularly if the diabetes is poorly controlled. Maternal systemic lupus erythematosus may be associated with congenital complete heart block.

If parents already have a child with congenital heart disease, the risk of recurrence is between 1 and 3% depending on the original lesion. If affected, siblings tend to have the same lesion or a similar one. There is also an increased incidence of heart defects in children of parents who were themselves born with congenital heart disease. There has recently been great improvement in prenatal detection, and fetal echocardiography can now detect most major heart defects at 18-weeks' gestation, so all high-risk mothers should be referred for this specialist screening.

Although there are a multitude of different congenital defects, 70–80% of cases are due to eight specific lesions. The commonest lesion is a ventricular septal defect (VSD) which accounts for a third of all cases.

Rather than give an exhaustive list of defects and their manifestations, we will take a management-based approach of cardiac problems in the newborn. Heart disease may be suspected when a baby exhibits certain symptoms. Equally, suspicion may be aroused by chance findings on routine examination of an asymptomatic baby. Only 40–50% of congenital heart disease is diagnosed by the first week of life, and 50–60% by 1 month.

The commonest congenital lesions that present in the first week of life are as follows:
• hypoplastic left heart syndrome;
• transposition of the great arteries;
• coarctation of the aorta;
• multiple major cardiac defects.
Presentation in the newborn falls into seven categories, some of which may be present at the same time.
1 Cyanosis.
2 Heart failure.
3 Heart murmur.
4 Impalpable femoral artery.
5 Abnormal heart rate.
6 Sudden hypotension.
7 The heart is on the wrong side.

THE BABY LOOKS BLUE

What does this mean?
A blue baby has cyanosis. The blue appearance is caused by an

excess of deoxygenated (reduced) haemoglobin in the blood, which in turn is due to a low oxygen saturation of the blood. The concentration of reduced haemoglobin must be at least 5 g/dl to give the appearance of cyanosis. The blue appearance depends on the proportion of desaturated haemoglobin as well as the haemoglobin level in the blood. Hence an anaemic baby will appear cyanosed less readily, whereas a polycythaemic baby may appear ruddy or cyanotic despite a normal arterial oxygen level.

Cyanosis is not always immediately apparent, and is particularly difficult to detect in dark-skinned babies. The colour is more a pale grey than blue. The cyanosis is said to be central when it affects the whole body, in particular the lips and tongue. Peripheral cyanosis refers to a blue colour of the hands and feet, most noticeable in the nail beds. Peripheral cyanosis is common in the newborn and is a normal finding in the first 48 hours. Central cyanosis however is *always* pathological and must be immediately investigated.

What is the underlying cause?

Having decided the baby has central cyanosis, the next thing to consider is the underlying cause.

Central cyanosis is usually due to cardiac or respiratory disease in the newborn. There are however other causes which must also be ruled out:

1 *Traumatic cyanosis* may occur when there is excessive delay between delivering the head and the trunk at birth. The face appears congested and bruised and petechiae are often present. The lips however remain pink and it resolves within a few days.

2 *Polycythaemia* may lead to a cyanotic appearance despite normal oxygen saturation levels, due to the high haemoglobin concentration (see p. 176).

3 *Pigmented skin.* Dark-skinned babies often appear to have cyanotic lips at birth; the tongue however, will be pink.

4 *Sepsis*, when severe, may lead to cyanosis, although it is usually peripheral due to poor peripheral circulation.

5 *Brain damage* from asphyxia or haemorrhage often causes cyanosis.

6 *Choanal atresia* when bilateral causes severe cyanosis and respiratory distress (see p. 104).

Respiratory vs cardiac disease

It is most important to differentiate between these causes of cyanosis. Any of the causes of respiratory distress discussed in Chapter 19 can lead to central cyanosis. The history may be helpful and pointers to respiratory disease include:

• prematurity (hyaline membrane disease);
• prolonged rupture of membranes (congenital pneumonia);
• meconium present at delivery (meconium aspiration);
• sudden deterioration in a ventilated baby (tension pneumothorax).

In general, babies with respiratory disease are more tachypnoeic and have more evident signs of respiratory distress (grunting, subcostal recession, nasal flaring) than babies with cardiac disease, particularly in the first 24–48 hours. An exception to this is when the baby has severe pulmonary oedema secondary to heart failure. Subcostal recession also occurs in congenital heart disease when there is increased pulmonary blood flow.

On examination there may be localizing signs in the chest that indicate pulmonary disease, although this is not usually very helpful. It must be stressed that a heart murmur is not always present in congenital heart disease, particularly in lesions causing cyanosis.

Sometimes a chest X-ray will be very helpful, even diagnostic if, for example, there is a pneumothorax or congenital diaphragmatic hernia. However in some conditions, X-ray signs are often non-specific at first, for example in hyaline membrane disease or congenital pneumonia.

The most useful investigation is an echocardiogram but this is not available in most hospitals. In this case, the hyperoxia test (also known as a nitrogen washout test) can be useful, particularly in helping to decide which babies should be referred for echocardiography. A disadvantage of the test is that it may induce closure of a patent ductus arteriosus which may cause deterioration of some babies with congenital heart disease. Some units have abandoned the test for this reason.

In pulmonary disease, either insufficient oxygen is reaching the lungs, or the alveoli are not being ventilated adequately so that oxygen does not diffuse through to the circulation. Hence if the inspired oxygen concentration is increased and the patient is ventilated optimally, the arterial oxygen concentration should also increase. On the other hand, in cyanotic heart disease, the oxygenated blood returning from the lungs never reaches the systemic circulation and it is deoxygenated blood returning from the body that is shunted back into the systemic circulation. So no matter how high the inspired oxygen concentration, the cyanosis will persist.

The baby should be given inspired oxygen at 95–100% concentration, either in a headbox or through the ventilator for 5–10 minutes. The baby's oxygen levels can be monitored using arterial blood samples or a transcutaneous oxygen monitor. The test should not be prolonged unnecessarily as an excessively high inspired oxygen concentration can damage the retina, particularly in premature babies. Results can be classified as follows:

- arterial P_{O_2} >20 kPa — respiratory disease probable;
- arterial P_{O_2} 13–20 kPa — cardiac disease likely;
- arterial P_{O_2} <13 kPa — cardiac disease probable.

Cyanotic heart disease
This results from cardiac lesions that divert deoxygenated blood returning from the body straight into the systemic circulation without first going to the lungs to pick up oxygen. This is known as a right-to-left shunt as blood returning to the 'right' side of the heart goes straight to the 'left' side of the heart and then out to the systemic circulation, thus bypassing the pulmonary circulation.

The principal lesions that present primarily with severe cyanosis in the newborn are:

- transposition of the great arteries (TGA) without adequate mixing of systemic and venous circulation;
- pulmonary atresia or severe pulmonary stenosis, which may or may not be accompanied by a ventricular septal defect;
- total anomalous pulmonary venous drainage (TAPVD) with obstruction to the venous return.

Transposition of the great arteries is the commonest of these conditions. The babies usually present within 24 hours of birth, and although cyanosed are otherwise well. Gradually however the baby becomes hypoxic and acidotic. If there are no other lesions, there will not be a heart murmur present. However if there is also a VSD, the cyanosis will appear later and the baby may present with heart failure. In addition the VSD will produce a heart murmur.

Tetralogy of Fallot is another major cause of cyanotic heart disease in childhood. It is not included in the above list as although it may occasionally present at birth, this is unusual and most infants develop cyanosis after a few months of life.

Full descriptions of all these anomalies will not be discussed here but can be found in many textbooks of paediatric heart disease.

The exact diagnosis will require echocardiography and perhaps cardiac catheterization at a specialist centre. There may be clues from the chest X-ray or electrocardiogram (ECG).

On the chest X-ray, the two things to look for, apart from the presence of primary lung disease, are:

1 Shape of the heart.
2 Vascularity of the lungs.

In TGA, the heart classically has a narrow pedicle and resembles an egg on its side. The lung fields are normal or there is increased vascularity. In pulmonary atresia, although there may be an enlarged right atrium, the heart essentially looks normal. However there will be reduced blood flow to the lungs so there are reduced vascular markings and the lungs look dark. In TAPVD, the heart looks relatively normal but here there is marked pulmonary venous congestion so the lungs have increased markings and look whiter.

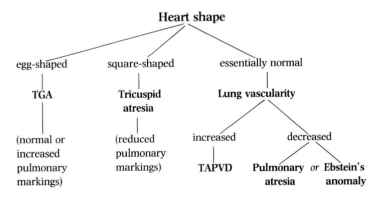

Once the diagnosis of cyanotic heart disease has been made, urgent referral is necessary, without delaying for further investigations apart from a chest X-ray.

Immediate management

In some cardiac conditions that cause cyanosis, blood can only reach the lungs through the ductus arteriosus which connects the aortic arch to the pulmonary artery. These babies will deteriorate once the ductus closes after birth and are said to have duct-dependent lesions. Examples are pulmonary atresia and transposition of the great arteries without a septal defect.

It is essential to keep the ductus arteriosus open until full assessment and diagnosis can be made at the cardiac centre. This can be achieved by giving an intravenous infusion of prostaglandin E_2. If the baby has a defect that is not duct-dependent, no harm will have been done by keeping the duct open temporarily. All babies with cyanotic heart disease should be given prostaglandin E_2 prior to transfer. It is however sensible to discuss this first with the referral centre.

The dose of prostaglandin E_2 given by continuous infusion ranges from 0.03 to 0.10 µg/kg/minute. For transferring the baby it is best to start at 0.05 µg/kg/minute. Ampoules of prostaglandin E_2 are 1 mg/ml. Add 1 ml to 500 ml 5% dextrose (giving a concentration of 2 µg/ml of prostaglandin E_2). An infusion of 0.05 µg/kg/minute is the same as 3 µg/kg/hour. Therefore to give an infusion of 0.05 µg/kg/minute, the solution should be given at 1.5 ml/kg/hour.

For example, a 3 kg baby would receive 1.5 × 3 = 4.5 ml/hour.

A potential side effect of the prostaglandin is apnoea, so it is safest to ventilate the baby for the journey. Other side effects sometimes seen are hypotension, pyrexia, muscle twitching and irritability. The use of prostaglandin has greatly improved the condition of these babies prior to surgery.

Attention should also be paid to the following prior to transfer:
• hypothermia must be prevented;
• metabolic acidosis should be corrected with bicarbonate;
• blood glucose and calcium must be corrected if abnormal.

It is safer to ventilate the babies for transfer if they are sick or on a prostaglandin infusion. It is sufficient to give the baby 30–40% oxygen; a higher oxygen concentration should be avoided as it may promote closure of the ductus arteriosus. Besides which, when there is a right-to-left shunt a high oxygen concentration will have little impact on the arterial oxygen level.

Persistent fetal circulation

This is a condition in which there is a persistence of the fetal haemodynamics after birth. The main effect is a high pulmonary vascular resistance so that there is pulmonary hypertension and the pressure in the pulmonary circulation is higher than that in the systemic circulation. The result is a right-to-left shunt through the ductus arteriosus and foramen ovale, leading to cyanosis and hypoxia.

The condition is associated with fetal distress and there is often a history of difficulty resuscitating the baby. It may also follow meconium aspiration, congenital pneumonia and pulmonary hypoplasia. The heart is normal apart from a secondary dilatation of the right atrium and ventricle due to pulmonary hypertension.

The baby presents within 24 hours of birth with respiratory distress and cyanosis. They are usually extremely unwell. The chest X-ray shows an enlarged heart with reduced vascular markings in the lungs. Giving the baby 100% oxygen does not improve the arterial oxygen level and the baby remains cyanosed. Echocardiography excludes congenital heart disease.

Treatment involves correcting any other abnormalities such as acidosis and hypoglycaemia. The baby will require mechanical ventilation. Drug therapy is aimed at reducing the pulmonary vascular resistance with vasodilators. Both tolazoline and prosta-cyclin infusions have been used, sometimes leading to a dramatic improvement. Neither drug is totally selective for the pulmonary vasculature so there is usually an accompanying fall in systemic blood pressure. Inotropic drugs such as dopamine may also be necessary. Despite intensive treatment, there is still a 30% mortality from this condition, and 50% of the survivors have some form of deafness although the reason is not clear.

THE BABY HAS SIGNS OF HEART FAILURE

Significance

Besides cyanosis, heart failure is the other main way that severe heart disease presents in the newborn. It may of course be present at the same time as cyanosis. The earlier the baby presents with signs of heart failure, the more serious the underlying condition. Any baby who develops heart failure within the first month will need immediate referral to a cardiologist for full investigation.

Presentation

The newborn tend to present with the following:

• tachycardia >180/minute, which may be accompanied by an obvious third heart sound loudest at the apex which causes a gallop rhythm;

• tachypnoea >60/minute;

• weight gain >30g/day despite poor feeding;

• hepatomegaly with the liver palpable more than 2 cm below the costal margin;

• fever and sweatiness due to a high metabolic rate, especially after feeds;

• cool extremities due to poor peripheral blood flow;

• peripheral oedema is rare in infants although periorbital oedema is sometimes seen.

In addition, if there is left ventricular failure with pulmonary oedema, there may be crepitations heard in the lungs or even a wheeze and the baby may have a dry cough. The heart is usually enlarged unless the failure is due to obstructed pulmonary venous return when it remains small. The chest X-ray usually shows an enlarged heart with increased vascular markings. The ECG will show evidence of right ventricular hypertrophy with right axis deviation.

Causes

The commonest congenital heart lesions causing heart failure are a ventricular septal defect (VSD) and a patent ductus arteriosus (PDA). However these rarely lead to heart failure in the first few weeks of life, apart from when they are found in premature babies. These two lesions will be discussed later.

Symptoms in the newborn are more likely due to more complex lesions. The following are some of the congenital heart defects that present primarily with heart failure in the newborn:

- hypoplastic left heart syndrome;
- coarctation of the aorta with or without a VSD;
- severe aortic stenosis;
- complex multiple defects.

There are other causes of heart failure in the newborn:

Myocardial ischaemia is occasionally seen in babies with birth asphyxia. Fetal hypoxia leads to a reduction in myocardial glycogen on which the heart is dependent for its supply of glucose. There may be ECG changes with ST depression and inverted T waves. Treatment of the failure leads to rapid improvement and the heart usually recovers well.

Hypoglycaemia itself can also lead to heart failure if the myocardium becomes depleted of glycogen.

Hypocalcaemia can lead to heart failure in the newborn which responds to treatment with IV calcium.

Systemic arteriovenous malformations are uncommon but if large can cause heart failure. The malformations are usually in the brain (e.g. aneurysm of the great vein of Galen) or the liver. There may be accompanying angiomas on the skin. Due to the large shunt of blood from artery to vein, the heart cannot keep up with the extra cardiac output required. A bruit may be heard over the skull or liver depending on the site of the malformation. Embolizing the feeding vessel surgically or radiologically is sometimes successful.

Iatrogenic IV fluid overload can occur if proper care is not taken, particularly in preterm babies.

Septicaemia may affect the heart if severe.

Treatment
Treatment of heart failure should be started before referral to a

specialist centre. Congenital heart disease that presents only with heart failure is unlikely to respond completely to medical management and surgery will usually be required. Treatment is as follows:

1 *Oxygen.* If unwell, the babies should receive 30% oxygen which should be humidified.

2 *Posture.* It may help the baby if he is nursed with his head raised by tilting the incubator tray.

3 *Feeding* should be given as small frequent feeds. The total fluid intake should be restricted to 120 ml/kg/day although it is important that adequate calories are given in view of the raised metabolic rate.

4 *Temperature control.* It is important that babies are not allowed to become overheated.

5 *Sedation* should be given if the baby is restless and distressed. Respiratory depressants should be avoided. Antihistamine sedatives such as trimeprazine (0.5–1.0 mg/kg 6 hourly) or promethazine (1 mg/kg 8 hourly) are suitable.

6 *Diuretics* are the mainstay of drug treatment. Frusemide is the drug of choice and can be given orally or intravenously if heart failure is severe or the baby is not tolerating oral fluids. Frusemide dose is 1–2 mg/kg 12 hourly. This can be increased to 2–4 mg/kg depending on the response. An alternative is to use a thiazide diuretic such as chlorothiazide for maintenance therapy. The dose is 20–30 mg/kg/day orally.

Plasma sodium and potassium must be monitored as hyponatraemia and hypokalaemia can result from increased electrolyte loss in the urine induced by the diuretics. Potassium supplements may be necessary (potassium chloride 2 mmol/kg/day) or a potassium-sparing diuretic such as amiloride or spironolactone can also be given.

7 *Inotropic drugs* may also be necessary. Digoxin is now used less often and the indications are less clear. It should be given under specialist supervision for certain cases only. It must be avoided in infants who have high pulmonary blood flow and severe left ventricular overload that results in a high cardiac output. It should also not be given to children with outflow tract obstruction such as tetralogy of Fallot. Digoxin levels must be monitored

and toxic levels are indicated by vomiting, diarrhoea and the development of certain arrhythmias (persistent bradycardia, atrioventricular dissociation or extrasystoles).

8 *Vasodilators* may sometimes be necessary and should be given only under specialist supervision. Captropril has been shown to be useful.

In addition, care must be taken to ensure that acidosis, hypoglycaemia, hypocalcaemia and anaemia are treated promptly or avoided in the first place.

THE BABY HAS A MURMUR

Heart murmurs are sounds caused by a disturbance of blood flow, usually because the flow has become turbulent. The loudness of the murmur is dependent on the pressure gradient as well as the volume of blood that is moving through the defect.

There is not always an abnormality present; sometimes the murmur is non-pathological or innocent. Innocent murmurs are common in childhood.

It is important for a junior paediatrician to recognize that there is a murmur present and alert a senior colleague. You are not expected to make the definitive diagnosis of the cardiac lesion.

Due to haemodynamic changes from the fetal circulation, murmurs may be heard in the first 24 hours or so that are not significant and never heard again. It is better to wait at least 24 hours before assessing the baby's heart at routine examination. In addition, certain defects that have characteristic murmurs once the circulation has settled, may not produce a murmur at first or it may be uncharacteristic. Among children who have a murmur from congenital heart disease heard at 2 years of age, only 20% have an audible murmur in the first week of life. Some congenital defects do not produce a murmur for many years (e.g. an atrial septal defect) whilst many lesions are associated with normal heart sounds.

A baby with a heart murmur may have one of the following:
• symptomatic cardiac defect;
• asymptomatic cardiac defect;
• normal heart.

Symptomatic cardiac defects

If a baby has symptomatic heart disease the presence of a murmur may provide more evidence that the problem really is cardiac. However the murmur itself is of less importance as it will already be obvious that the child will need cardiac imaging for a diagnosis to be made.

Most babies with cyanotic heart disease do not have a heart murmur. For example, transposition of the great arteries will only be associated with a murmur if there is also a ventricular septal defect present.

Acyanotic heart disease is usually due to abnormal communications through the atrial or ventricular walls or at the aortopulmonary level. The pressures remain normal, with pressure on the left side of the heart being greater than that on the right side of the heart. Hence blood will flow through the defect from left to right, which is known as a left-to-right shunt. The extra turbulence set up by this type of flow will result in a murmur, which is usually heard during the systolic part of the cardiac cycle. Examples of this type of defect are atrial septal defect (ASD), ventricular septal defect (VSD), atrioventricular canal defects and patent ductus arteriosus (PDA). These defects are not always symptomatic.

Acyanotic heart disease may also be due to obstruction to flow within the heart or major vessels that is not associated with abnormal communications. Blood will flow in the right direction but the tight valve will produce turbulent flow and a heart murmur. Examples of this type of defect are pulmonary or aortic stenosis. The murmurs are also usually systolic and will be loudest over the affected area. Many of these cases are asymptomatic unless the lesion is severe.

Asymptomatic cardiac defects

A heart murmur may be detected on routine examination of a perfectly well baby. It may be first heard at the initial examination, but as mentioned earlier, due to the haemodynamic changes, it may not be picked up until the 6-week check or later still. The main issue in these cases is to decide whether there is an underlying defect or whether the murmur is innocent. This is dealt with later.

The main asymptomatic lesions that are associated with a murmur are:

• small ventricular septal defect — loud pansystolic murmur at left sternal edge;

• patent ductus arteriosus — continuous murmur (systolic and diastolic) loudest under left clavicle;

• pulmonary stenosis — harsh ejection systolic murmur over pulmonary area;

• aortic stenosis — ejection systolic murmur over aortic area.

Clearly the outlook depends on the underlying lesion and this varies greatly. In the case of a small VSD or PDA, the defect is of little significance and the parents can be reassured. If the diagnosis is confirmed then follow-up will not be necessary.

The prognosis for pulmonary and aortic stenosis is not so certain. Most cases of mild pulmonary stenosis have an excellent outlook. Aortic stenosis on the other hand has a tendency to progress in severity. These cases will need to be followed up by a cardiologist.

Tetralogy of Fallot leads to cyanosis in most infants by 6 months, and without corrective surgery most patients will die before 20–25 years, the average being about 5 years of age.

Two of the congenital defects that have been mentioned are so common that they warrant further discussion.

Ventricular septal defect
This is the commonest congenital lesion and accounts for about a third of the defects that present in childhood. There is usually only one hole between the two ventricles but they can be multiple. The size varies and they are classified as small, medium and large.

Small defects account for about 70% of cases and the child is asymptomatic. There is an insignificant left-to-right shunt and usually a loud pansystolic murmur best heard over the left fourth intercostal space. There may also be a palpable thrill. Most of these defects close spontaneously and the murmur disappears. In some the defect remains but becomes so small that it is clinically insignificant.

Medium and large defects lead to a large left-to-right shunt and so there is a long loud systolic murmur with a diastolic flow murmur at the apex. If the defect is very large, the pressure in the two ventricles becomes the same. However blood still flows from left to right as the vascular resistance is lower in the pulmonary vessels than in the systemic ones. Without surgical correction, eventually the pulmonary vascular resistance increases and the shunt decreases or even reverses so the murmur disappears. Infants with large defects present with heart failure after 3 weeks of life. The larger defects will not respond to medical treatment and require surgery to control heart failure and prevent pulmonary hypertension. Overall, 20% of cases of isolated VSD need surgical closure, usually within the first 2 years of life.

Patent ductus arteriosus
In the fetus, the ductus arteriosus takes blood from the pulmonary artery to the aorta, bypassing the lungs. At birth, the duct closes within 10–15 hours. Sometimes however the duct remains open, and this is particularly common in preterm babies. Blood then flows from the aorta to the lower pressure pulmonary artery causing a left-to-right shunt.

A small defect is usually noted on routine examination and is asymptomatic. A continuous murmur is noted, heard loudest just below the left clavicle. Larger defects will present with signs of heart failure after the first month. The murmur may be limited to the systolic phase and there are bounding pulses. Preterm babies often show non-specific signs and there may be difficulty weaning them off the ventilator.

A PDA usually closes spontaneously in preterm babies and closure can still occur within the first 3 months. However sometimes treatment is necessary if the baby is symptomatic. Initially fluids are restricted to 120 ml/kg/day and 30% oxygen given (hypoxia keeps the duct open). If this is not effective, closure is often achieved by giving 1–3 doses of indomethacin. Otherwise surgery is necessary which involves a very simple procedure.

In fullterm babies, spontaneous closure is uncommon and will not occur after 2 weeks of life. If the lesion is small and the child asymptomatic, treatment is not immediately necessary, although there is always a risk of bacterial endarteritis. Surgery is usually recommended for most infants.

Infective endocarditis

Turbulent blood flow at the site of a cardiac defect can give rise to damage to the endocardial lining of the heart. There is then a risk of bacteria adhering to the damaged area and causing infective endocarditis. The risk of infection depends on the lesion and is highest when a jet of blood passes at high velocity through a narrow hole, for example a small ventricular septal defect or stenosis of an aortic valve. Endocarditis is rare under 2 years of age but all children with a cardiac lesion, including those with asymptomatic lesions, must be given antibiotic prophylaxis when undergoing dental procedures or gastrointestinal and genitourinary surgery. Details of suitable antibiotic regimes for prophylaxis are available in the *British National Formulary*. In addition, advice should be given to the parents about dental hygiene and the child should have regular dental checks. Fluoride supplementation is advisable if the child lives in an area where the water has a low fluoride content.

Innocent murmurs in a normal heart

Innocent murmurs are physiological murmurs that are heard in the normal heart or great vessels. They are also known as flow or functional murmurs. They are common and most children will have a murmur when tachycardic.

There are certain features that point to a murmur being benign:
• the child is asymptomatic;
• the murmur is short and soft;
• the murmur is heard over a limited area rather than over the whole cardiac area;
• the murmur varies with posture;
• the murmur is louder when the baby is tachycardic from whatever cause (e.g. fever, crying);
• there are no other abnormal cardiac signs;
• chest X-ray and ECG are normal.

Despite these clues, the diagnosis of an innocent murmur is not always straightforward and if there is any doubt the infant should be referred to a cardiologist. Normal echocardiography will confirm the diagnosis. The parents can be reassured but often

Table 20.1 Cardiac defects in the newborn that do not produce a murmur.

Cyanotic	Acyanotic
Transposition of the great arteries	Coarctation of the aorta
Total anomalous pulmonary venous drainage with an obstruction	Cor triatrium
Hypoplastic left heart syndrome	Myocarditis
Pulmonary atresia ± ventricular septal defect	
Tricuspid atresia	

find it difficult to accept the child's heart is normal when they are aware of the murmur.

The murmur heard on postnatal routine examination
If the baby is otherwise well and asymptomatic the child should be seen in clinic in 2–4 weeks. If the murmur is still present (and many have resolved by then) a chest X-ray and ECG should be done and the baby should be referred to a cardiologist. Should the baby develop symptoms at any stage further investigation and urgent referral are necessary.

The abnormal heart with no murmur
Many cardiac defects do not produce a murmur in the newborn (Table 20.1).

THE BABY HAS AN IMPALPABLE FEMORAL ARTERY

An important part of routine examination of the newborn is to feel for pulsation in both femoral arteries. This is often difficult, especially if the baby is moving or crying. However if the femoral pulses are impalpable, the diagnosis of coarctation of the aorta must be considered.

Coarctation refers to a narrowing in the aorta adjacent to

where the ductus arteriosus joins the aorta. It is probably due to some specialized ductal contractile tissue spreading during development to form a band around the aorta.

Mild cases may be asymptomatic but the femoral pulses will be absent or difficult to feel. In contrast, the right arm pulses will be easily felt. The left arm pulses will be normal unless the left subclavian is also involved in the coarctation.

If there is any doubt, the baby should have the blood pressure measured in all four limbs by the Dinamap doppler machine. The pressure in the upper limbs should not be more than 15–20 mmHg higher than that in the lower limbs. If the diagnosis is still suspected, the baby must be urgently referred to a cardiology centre.

Severe coarctation of the aorta usually presents in the first 2 weeks and the timing of presentation is dependent on closure of the ductus arteriosus. Once the duct has closed completely, blood can only enter the descending aorta to reach the lower half of the body through the tight coarctation. Left ventricular failure develops and poor blood flow to the kidney, liver and gut lead to oliguria, acidosis, hypoglycaemia and hypocalcaemia. The babies often collapse and may be extremely ill.

A prostaglandin E_2 infusion will open the ductus arteriosus and should lead to improvement. Vigorous treatment with dopamine and diuretics may also be necessary. Urgent referral is needed for immediate surgery. The long-term outlook depends on the presence of other cardiac lesions, as over half the cases have associated defects, particularly ventricular septal defects, aortic stenosis and mitral valve disease. Without surgery, severe coarctation is fatal.

THE BABY HAS AN ABNORMAL HEART RATE

The normal heart rate in the newborn is 110–160 beats/minute. Outside this range, the baby is tachycardic (fast) or bradycardic (slow).

Tachycardia
Tachycardia is uncommon in babies. A heart rate over 180/

minute usually indicates the presence of heart failure. Anaemic babies may also be tachycardic.

A heart rate over 200/minute may be due to a supraventricular tachycardia which is unusual in the newborn. The baby may be asymptomatic but can present with sudden collapse or a gradual onset of heart failure (see p. 235).

Bradycardia

Transient bradycardia commonly accompanies apnoeic episodes in premature babies (see p. 213). Sometimes the bradycardia is noticed before the baby becomes apnoeic.

Bradycardia can also be induced iatrogenically due to vagal stimulation. This happens with overvigorous pharyngeal suction or with clumsy intubation.

Persistent bradycardia may be due to congenital complete heart block. Sometimes the bradycardia is first detected at delivery and a false diagnosis of fetal distress is made which may lead to an unnecessary emergency Caesarean section. The baby may develop heart failure or ectopic beats in which case referral to a cardiologist is necessary.

THE BABY HAS COLLAPSED
WITH SUDDEN HYPOTENSION

Sometimes a baby presents with a sudden severe collapse which may be of cardiac origin. The following are some of the possible causes:

Closure of ductus arteriosus in a duct-dependent lesion. When systemic blood flow is dependent on passage through the ductus, if the duct closes the child may collapse with cardiogenic shock. Examples of these sorts of defects are severe coarctation of the aorta, critical aortic stenosis, aortic atresia and an interrupted aortic arch. Hypoplastic left heart syndrome may also be duct-dependent.

Duct-dependent pulmonary blood flow will lead to severe cyanosis rather than sudden collapse when the duct closes. Keeping the duct open with prostaglandin E_2 should lead to improvement in the short term.

Arrhythmias. Supraventricular tachycardia (SVT) can sometimes present with sudden collapse. It may be possible to abort the arrhythmia by stimulating the baby's vagus nerve. This is best achieved by immersing the baby's face under ice-cold water briefly or applying an ice-pack to the face. Another method is to apply gentle pressure to the eyeballs but extreme care must be taken not to damage the eyes. If this does not work, the baby will need drug therapy or DC cardioversion.

Myocardial disease. Severe myocardial ischaemia following birth asphyxia may sometimes present with collapse and shock. The baby has poor peripheral circulation and metabolic acidosis. The chest X-ray will show cardiomegaly with venous congestion and pulmonary oedema.

Acute myocarditis can also present with sudden collapse. The cause is usually viral, due to either Coxsackie B or ECHO virus. There is often a prodromal phase of vomiting and lethargy. After a few days, the infant becomes breathless or suddenly collapses with cardiogenic shock (tachycardia with poor peripheral pulses, tachypnoea, cyanosis and a mottled appearance, hypotension, large liver). Chest X-ray shows mild cardiomegaly with obvious pulmonary venous congestion and often interstitial oedema. ECG shows low voltage QRS complexes with flat T waves and a prolonged Q–T interval. There may also be large or wide P waves. Treatment involves diuretics and often a dopamine infusion is also necessary. One third of cases with cardiogenic shock die despite treatment and only half the infants make a complete recovery.

Hypoplastic left heart syndrome. The whole left side of the heart is underdeveloped. The baby often becomes extremely ill within a few hours of birth, and certainly within a few days. They usually seem normal at birth, but during the first day become breathless and slightly blue. When the ductus arteriosus closes, they rapidly deteriorate and heart failure develops. If a murmur is present at all, it is a faint systolic murmur heard best at the left sternal edge. Sometimes the initial presentation is with sudden collapse and severe acidosis that has no obvious cause. The baby is usually thought to have septicaemia. The condition is invariably fatal unless heart transplant is possible. Recently a palliative operation has been devised but results so far have not been encouraging.

THE BABY'S HEART IS ON THE WRONG SIDE

Dextrocardia refers to a heart that is not in the normal position but is in the right side of the chest with its apex pointing to the patient's right. However dextrocardia is often used as a broad term which includes a heart that is displaced to the right side by pulmonary disease or is rotated. More correctly a heart that is anatomically on the wrong side is said to be 'malpositioned'.

When the heart is malpositioned in the right thorax, the abdominal organs are also usually on the wrong side, with the liver on the left and the stomach on the right (situs inversus of the abdominal viscera).

Dextrocardia may be noticed on routine examination by careful palpation of the apex beat. Listening to the heart, especially in small babies is not always helpful as heart sounds are loud throughout the chest. Sometimes the diagnosis is a chance finding on X-ray.

An abdominal X-ray is necessary to look for the stomach bubble to identify the position of the abdominal viscera. Echocardiography is also necessary as there may be associated cardiac abnormalities. If the heart is otherwise normal, then there are no physiological effects.

INVESTIGATING CARDIAC DISEASE

Echocardiography is now the most important investigation for diagnosing cardiac defects. It is essentially an ultrasound examination and is safe and non-invasive, so can easily be used on sick infants. The anatomical structures of the heart and major vessels can be clearly delineated. In addition, Doppler echocardiography with colour flow imaging will show the direction and speed of blood flow within the heart.

Because of the advances in echocardiography, cardiac catheterization is now used less often, particularly in babies. This advance is fortunate as catheterization can be a risky procedure in sick neonates and often causes a deterioration in their condition. Cardiac catheterization involves inserting a long hollow radio-opaque catheter into the heart and great vessels, via a large peripheral artery or vein usually in the groin or antecubital fossa. Pressures and oxygen saturation can be measured in the various sites. In addition, by inserting contrast medium anatomical structures can be further delineated.

TREATMENT OF CONGENITAL DEFECTS

Over half the children with congenital heart disease require some type of surgery. Operations tend to be palliative or corrective. Palliative operations are usually carried out when the baby is too small or sick to have major correction, or when a corrective procedure does not exist. Some of these operations may give long-term symptom relief even though the defect has not been fully corrected.

One of the commonest procedures is to insert a shunt in the form of a Gore-Tex tube between a systemic artery and one of the pulmonary arteries. This increases pulmonary blood flow and reduces cyanosis. The modified Blalock–Taussig shunt connects the right subclavian artery to the right pulmonary artery. Artificial shunts produce a loud harsh systolic murmur.

The other common procedure is pulmonary banding. Infants who have complex defects that lead to high pulmonary blood flow with a high pulmonary artery pressure can have a piece of tape tied round the pulmonary artery to form an artificial constriction. This reduces the flow and the pressure beyond the level of the banding.

Some procedures can now be performed without direct access to the heart, using catheterization techniques. Balloons have been used to dilate valve stenoses (valvuloplasty) as well as stenosed major vessels. The procedures are still new and await long-term evaluation. Holes can also be produced in the atrial septa (septostomy) either by using a balloon catheter or a blade inserted via a catheter. This is known as the Rashkind procedure and offers immediate palliation for certain conditions such as transposition of the great arteries.

Corrective operations tend to be more complex and dangerous, except for closure of a patent ductus arteriosus which is relatively simple. Cardiopulmonary bypass is necessary for most open-heart surgery. New procedures are continually being devised and the mortality figures are gradually improving. The risks tend to be related to the actual defect and whether it is correctable.

Ultimately the only option for some complex defects may be a heart transplant or a heart–lung transplant. Mortality is high although it has improved with the immunosuppressant agent, cyclosporin. The main problem is still the short supply of donor organs, particularly for the newborn.

FURTHER READING

Jordan SC & Scott O (1988) *Heart Disease in Paediatrics.* Butterworth, London.
Gillette PC (1990) Congenital heart disease. *Pediatric Clinics of North America* 37(1): 1–239.

21: Convulsions

RECOGNITION

Recognition of a neonatal convulsion is not always obvious as it is sometimes difficult to distinguish normal and abnormal movements in the newborn. The added difficulty is that the convulsion has usually ceased by the time the baby is seen and often the only evidence is the description.

Neonatal convulsions tend to be repetitive jerky movements (clonic seizure) which may be generalized or restricted to one or more limbs. When the fit is localized (focal) the baby usually remains fully conscious. Focal fits may start in one part of the body and shift to another part. Another form, seen more often in preterm babies, is a generalized stiffening of the body. The limbs are held in rigid extension (tonic seizure) that resembles the decerebrate posture. Another type of seizure is manifest by rapid

isolated jerks (myoclonic seizure). Although commoner in premature babies it occasionally occurs in fullterm babies. Myoclonic
seizures tend to indicate a severe insult to the brain.

The fit may be subtle and witnesses may not realize that the
baby has just had a convulsion. Manifestations of a fit may
include deviation of the eyes to one side, rapid blinking of the
eyes or fluttering of the eyelids, lip smacking and sucking,
quivering or odd tongue movements, cycling movements of the
legs, or simply an apnoeic episode.

Fits may or may not be accompanied by loss of consciousness
or apnoea. Sometimes the convulsion itself was not witnessed but
apnoea or a transient cyanotic episode may indicate that a fit has
occurred.

CAUSES

Just over 1% of neonates have a convulsion and there are many
causes. However over 90% of cases are due to the following:
• injury to the brain;
• hypoglycaemia;
• hypocalcaemia ($\pm$ hypomagnesaemia);
• meningitis.
Other causes will be dealt with later.

Injury to the brain

Anoxia and ischaemia are the commonest causes of damage to
the brain and may occur before, during or after delivery. Hypoxia
reduces the amount of oxygen available to the brain for metabolism and causes profound biochemical changes. Ischaemia
decreases cerebral blood perfusion and may lead to infarction of
brain tissue. Hypoxic-ischaemic encephalopathy is the commonest cause of neonatal convulsions. The fits are seen early,
sometimes within 2–12 hours of birth in an asphyxiated baby.
When convulsions start even earlier, the implication is that the
hypoxic insult occurred some time before delivery. The fits are
usually frequent and severe, they may even be continuous.

Intracranial haemorrhage due to birth injury is less common
and is often associated with rapid delivery of a preterm infant.

The fits tend to occur on the second day and are usually focal. Subdural haemorrhage, which is associated with larger babies, is now rarely seen.

Intracranial haemorrhage, unrelated to birth injury, commonly occurs in sick preterm babies (see p. 122). If severe it may lead to convulsions. Subarachnoid haemorrhage may present with a convulsion in a premature baby who is otherwise well, usually on the second day of life.

Hypoglycaemia

Along with complications of birth, hypoglycaemia is the other main cause of convulsions that presents early, usually within the first day or two. Neurological symptoms of hypoglycaemia are commoner in small babies as opposed to the large infants of diabetic mothers. Hypoglycaemia is dealt with in Chapter 14.

Hypocalcaemia

Hypocalcaemia is considered to be the cause of a convulsion if the serum calcium is below 1.75 mmol/l, although symptoms are unusual unless the level is below 1.5 mmol/l. However not all babies with hypocalcaemia are symptomatic and hypocalcaemia may be present in babies who have another cause for the convulsion.

Hypocalcaemia that occurs in the first 2–3 days is usually associated with low birthweight infants, particularly babies who are small-for-dates (see p. 126). It may also be associated with birth asphyxia. In these cases, the low serum calcium is not usually the prime cause of the convulsions. Hypocalcaemia may be found in any sick baby due to the stress response which causes high blood levels of glucocorticoids and calcitonin. Infants of diabetic mothers are also prone to hypocalcaemia.

Late hypocalcaemia may be seen at the end of the first week and causes neonatal tetany. This is manifest by jitteriness, clonus of the jaw, knee or ankle and focal seizures. Late hypocalcaemia is almost unknown in breastfed babies, and is extremely rare in bottle-fed babies now that the infant formula milks are modified to be close to human milk.

Hypocalcaemia may be associated with a low serum magnesium of less than 0.6 mmol/l. Although rare, hypomagnesaemia may also cause neonatal tetany without accompanying hypocalcaemia.

Another uncommon cause of hypocalcaemia is maternal vitamin D deficiency that is found in certain ethnic groups who are at risk of developing rickets.

Meningitis

Meningitis may lead to convulsions but this is a late sign and the baby does not usually first present with a fit (see p. 187). Septicaemia and any severe infection can cause convulsions.

Other causes

Once the above causes are excluded, other less common causes must be considered. We will not give an exhaustive list but will mention some of the more likely possibilities.

Sodium imbalance. Hyponatraemia may lead to jitteriness followed by extensor tonic fits. It may arise if a baby is overloaded with hypo-osmolar IV fluids, after vigorous treatment of hypoglycaemia for example, with glucose solutions that do not contain sodium chloride. Overhydration is also more likely in babies who have meningitis or intracranial haemorrhage as cerebral insult often leads to inappropriate ADH secretion with resulting water retention.

Hypernatraemia may be associated with dehydration although this is uncommon as babies with diarrhoea and vomiting more commonly have a low or normal serum sodium. It can also arise from adding too much milk powder to the water when making up a formula feed. Hypernatraemia can lead to clonic fits.

Polycythaemia can cause fits secondary to cerebral venous thrombosis if the packed cell volume is very high (see p. 176).

Drug withdrawal in babies whose mothers take narcotics through pregnancy is an increasing problem (see p. 9). 10–20% of the babies have clonic fits. Maternal use of barbiturates and excessive alcohol are also associated with convulsions.

Structural abnormalities of the brain are responsible for less than 5% of neonatal convulsions.

Congenital infections such as cytomegalovirus and toxoplasmosis can present with fits (see pp. 19 and 23).

Inborn errors of metabolism are rare, but disorders of amino acid metabolism, particularly maple syrup urine disease may present with neonatal seizures. Other features that may be present are lethargy or stupor, hypotonia, food intolerance and the baby may have a peculiar smell.

Pyridoxine (vitamin B_6) deficiency is another rare cause of fits but is important as it is easily diagnosed and treated. If 50 mg pyridoxine is given intravenously during the fit, the convulsion will stop within a few minutes. Alternatively oral pyridoxine (100 mg/day) for 3 days will control the fits. It is worthwhile giving pyridoxine to any neonate who is having fits without an obvious cause. If the diagnosis is confirmed, vitamin B_6 supplements will be required for life.

Kernicterus. Although uncommon nowadays, severe hyperbilirubinaemia may lead to kernicterus and convulsions, particularly in sick preterm babies (see p. 169).

Familial neonatal convulsions is a rare disorder in which the baby has refractory fits, usually presenting on the second or third day. This may occur in several generations of the family and it is thought to have an autosomal dominant inheritance. If the baby does not suffer secondary hypoxia from the convulsions, recovery is complete and development is normal, although 14% of cases go on to develop epilepsy in later life.

No known cause is found in 3% of neonatal convulsions despite extensive investigations. A syndrome has been described called 'fifth-day fits' in which the baby has multifocal convulsions or apnoeic seizures that start on the fourth or fifth day of life. There is no known aetiology although a metabolic cause is postulated. The fits do not recur and development is normal.

INVESTIGATIONS

Investigations of a neonatal fit can be put into three categories: immediate, early and late.

Immediate — these are done at the time of the fit as the results may influence immediate management:
• blood glucose should be measured on a BM stix whilst the baby is still convulsing as IV glucose will be the treatment for the fit if the baby is hypoglycaemic;
• blood is also taken at the time the IV cannula is inserted and should be sent to the laboratory urgently to measure: plasma glucose, serum sodium and potassium, serum calcium, packed cell volume, venous pH, base excess and bicarbonate.

Early — these investigations should be performed once the baby has stopped fitting and may give clues to the aetiology;
• full blood count for white cell count and cell differential;
• blood culture;
• lumbar puncture (this is not always necessary, for example if the baby was hypoglycaemic and there are no other indications of sepsis);
• cranial ultrasound through the anterior fontanelle.

Late — these are not always necessary and would be done if fits were recurrent and aetiology had not been established:
• serum magnesium, particularly if the baby was also hypocalcaemic but the fits did not respond to calcium supplements:
• urine for amino acid chromatography;
• urine for drug screen (toxicology);
• examination of the child with an ultraviolet Wood's lamp which will show up any areas of depigmented skin that may be found in tuberose sclerosis (this is a syndrome of epilepsy, mental retardation, white or pale skin patches and the later development of an adenoma sebaceum rash on the face);
• CT (computerized tomography) scan is sometimes helpful;
• MRI (magnetic resonance imaging) scans are particularly useful for showing up subtle structural abnormalities of the brain;

• EEG (electroencephalography) may be indicated but is not always helpful. Between fits, minor EEG abnormalities are common but not always easy to interpret and a normal EEG does not necessarily rule out an abnormality in the brain. An EEG performed at the time of an abnormal movement may help determine whether this is a subtle seizure movement or simply benign. 24-hour EEGs that record the information can also sometimes be useful to confirm whether a baby is having fits in the first place;

• Video recordings of the baby may also be helpful in characterizing the type of fit if they have not been witnessed by medical staff. Synchronous video and EEG recordings can be very helpful but this is only available in some specialist neurology centres.

TREATMENT

First aid

It may be necessary to intubate and ventilate the baby if there is a prolonged apnoea, bradycardia or cyanosis. In any event oxygen should be given via a face mask for the duration of the fit.

It may also be necessary to suction the baby's mouth and oropharynx if the baby has vomited to prevent inhalation of stomach contents.

Treating the cause

In certain cases, treating the cause will also treat the convulsion.

Hypoglycaemia must be treated with a bolus of IV 10% glucose (5 ml/kg) followed by a 10% glucose infusion (see p. 164). If possible, milk should also be given once the fit has stopped.

Hypocalcaemia is treated with IV calcium if the baby is still fitting. Give 1 ml/kg of 10% calcium gluconate over 2–3 minutes. You must be certain that the IV cannula is properly sited in a large vein. Calcium causes severe burns if the cannula has 'tissued' and calcium is injected into the skin. The baby's heart rate must be monitored with a cardiorater while the IV calcium is given and the injection must be stopped if the baby becomes bradycardic. Hypocalcaemia is not as dangerous as hypoglycaemia so it is usually sufficient to give the calcium orally. 5–10 ml of 10% calcium gluconate per day added to the feeds is usually sufficient to correct the serum calcium level within 1–2 days.

Hypomagnesaemia is treated with 0.2 ml/kg of 50% magnesium sulphate given intramuscularly. This can be repeated after 6 hours if necessary but serum magnesium should be checked before a second dose is given. Occasionally the IM magnesium makes the baby hypotonic but this is reversed by giving calcium gluconate.

Pyridoxine deficiency has been mentioned earlier, and all fitting babies should receive 50 mg IV pyridoxine if the cause of the fit is not immediately apparent.

Treatment of other underlying causes should also be initiated but anticonvulsant therapy will also be required. Management of birth asphyxia is discussed on p. 36 and meningitis on p. 187.

Anticonvulsant therapy

This should be initiated if the fit lasts more than 3 minutes as prolonged fits can lead to hypoxia, hypertension and raised intracranial pressure. However it may be better not to give anticonvulsants for brief infrequent fits.

If the baby is having a fit, give 1 ml paraldehyde. If the baby is thin then this should be given rectally but if he is chubby then it can be given intramuscularly. The rectal paraldehyde should be mixed with an equal volume of arachis oil.

A second drug is given to prevent further fits. The first choice is phenytoin. There has been concern expressed over its possible adverse effects on cerebellar development but it is safe in the short-term. Give a loading dose of 15–20 mg/kg intravenously. It must be given slowly, over 15–20 minutes otherwise it can cause cardiac arrhythmias. The alternate drug is phenobarbitone and a loading dose of 15–20 mg/kg is given intravenously.

After this, an infusion of chlormethiazole 0.8% can be tried although it may involve large volumes of fluid. The dose starts at

0.6 ml/kg/hour and may be increased every 2–4 hours up to 2.25 ml/kg/hour depending on the response. However 0.6–1.25 ml/kg/hour is usually sufficient.

All anticonvulsants may cause a degree of respiratory depression so babies must be carefully monitored as artificial ventilation may be needed. Diazepam is not recommended for control of neonatal seizures.

Maintenance therapy

This is usually given to most babies. However some units wait to see whether fits recur before starting maintenance therapy as often babies only fit after an acute insult which may be transient and no longer relevant by the time the loading dose has worn off.

Phenytoin or phenobarbitone is given as an oral dose of 5 mg/kg once a day.

Depending on the cause of the fits, the drug is usually stopped after 7–10 days if the baby has remained fit-free and is well. In certain conditions, maintenance therapy is continued long-term. These include severe birth asphyxia, meningitis and malformations of the brain.

PROGNOSIS

This largely depends on the aetiology although generally convulsions that occur in the first few days carry a worse outlook. The worse progonsis is found with malformations of the brain or when the baby has persisting neurological abnormalities. Prognosis should be guarded when fits are secondary to severe birth asphyxia, intracranial haemorrhage (particularly if intracerebral), prolonged hypoglycaemia or meningitis.

The type of fit may also be a guide. Worse prognosis is found with tonic, myoclonic and subtle seizures as these tend to be associated with diffuse brain insults.

The EEG performed between fits may be helpful as a normal interictal EEG is associated with normal development in 86% of cases whereas multifocal abnormalities are associated with normal development in only 12% of cases.

JITTERY BABIES

Some babies are jittery and this must be distinguished from a true fit. In addition jitteriness may be physiological and perfectly benign.

Jitteriness refers to movements in a baby that are fast (10/second) and rhythmic with equal amplitude, which contrasts with the slower jerking movement of a fit which has a fast and slow component. The jitteriness is also easily provoked by any stimulus. In addition, the jittery movement of the limb can usually be stopped by flexing the limb which would have no effect in a fitting baby. Jittery babies also have normal eye movements whereas fits are often accompanied by deviation of the gaze.

Jitteriness may be a physiological finding and is common in small-for-dates babies. If the jitteriness stops when the baby sucks on a finger then it is usually benign. Should the jitteriness continue then causes should be sought. Common associated conditions are mild birth asphyxia, hypocalcaemia, hypoglycaemia and drug withdrawal. In persistent jitteriness it is worth checking the following:

- blood glucose;
- serum calcium;
- packed cell volume.

If there is no underlying cause, treatment is not necessary and the jitteriness usually settles after a feed.

FURTHER READING

O'Donohoe NV (1985) *Epilepsies of Childhood.* Butterworth, London.
Pellock JM, (1989) Seizure disorders, *Pediatric Clinics of North America,* **36**(2): 265–469.

22: Practical Procedures

Procedures on babies can be daunting for the inexperienced. You must never be afraid or too proud to ask for help from senior colleagues. It is better for an experienced doctor to supervise a procedure from the beginning than to be called later to a situation with fraught parents, doctor and baby.

A few general points should be made:
• always have everything ready before you start;
• explain everything carefully to the parents before beginning — including the reason for doing the test;
• ask the parents if they want to be present during the procedure as many of them will want to see what is happening to their baby;
• always ask a nurse to assist you, and if it is an intricate procedure such as a lumbar puncture ask for an experienced nurse;
• wash and dry your hands properly before starting any procedure;
• if you are having difficulty, call for help.

Certain procedures have not been included in this chapter as they are only performed on a neonatal intensive care unit, for example, inserting an umbilical artery catheter or performing ventricular taps. We have not included inserting chest drains although the emergency procedure for draining a tension pneumothorax is described on p. 55. There are many textbooks of neonatal intensive care that describe these procedures in detail.

All the procedures outlined below are described for the right-handed.

COLLECTING BLOOD SPECIMENS

Capillary blood samples
Small amounts of blood can be collected from the baby's heel. This is suitable for:
• capillary blood gases;
• blood glucose by BM stix method;
• serum bilirubin measured on a bilirubinometer;
• blood spots for the Guthrie card (see Appendix 6).

Larger samples (up to 1 ml) can be collected this way if there is no alternative. It is not ideal as it may lead to inaccuracies. Serum potassium is often too high due to the inevitable haemolysis that occurs with the heel-prick method. The packed cell volume is up to 15% higher than the true venous PCV. *Never* use this method for blood cultures. You will need:

- alcohol swab;
- sterile Vaseline;
- lancet;
- sample tube or capillary tube;
- cotton-wool balls;
- tape.

The heel must be warm, otherwise blood flow is poor. Warm it in your hand (which of course you have already washed) or put a cotton-wool ball soaked in warm water against the heel for a few minutes. Clean the heel with an alcohol swab and allow this to dry. Put a thin smear of vaseline from an unopened sterile tube on the heel. This will allow the blood to form proper drops that can be collected otherwise it runs off the heel in a fine streak.

The heel should be held in the left hand with the baby's ankle flexed (Fig. 22.1). Do not squeeze it so tightly that the heel goes

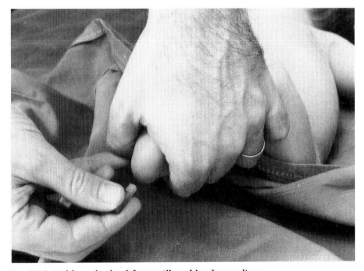

Fig. 22.1 Holding the heel for capillary blood sampling.

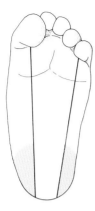

Fig. 22.2 Capillary blood sampling from a heel-prick (sample from the shaded areas only).

white or you will never obtain any blood. Squeeze it enough so that the heel is flushed red. Insert the lancet 1–2 mm into the skin. You can see from the diagram (Fig. 22.2) that it is the lateral fleshy portion of the heel that is punctured. Never prick the heel in the midline as you risk causing osteomyelitis in the os calcis (heel bone). Jabbing the bone is also extremely painful. If repeated samples are necessary vary the site used.

Be firm with your heel-prick and you will get a good sample of free-flowing blood. A tiny jab is not kinder to the baby as the blood does not come easily and you spend 5–10 minutes squeezing the heel. This is much more unpleasant for the baby than a swift proper heel-prick which is over in a matter of seconds.

Once the blood is collected, apply pressure to the bleeding area with a cotton-wool ball for a few minutes. The cotton-wool can be taped over the heel with thin papertape. This is better than using small elastoplasts as these are difficult to remove later.

Capillary blood gas estimations may be obtained from blood obtained by heel-prick. It is important to ensure a free-flowing sample is taken. Use the long heparinized capillary tubes and always take a spare sample as blood gas analysers sometimes swallow the samples without giving a result. There should be no air bubbles in the tube otherwise the sample is spoiled. The sample should be taken quickly to the blood gas analyser which you must be shown how to use. This expensive equipment is easily broken if used incorrectly, particularly if unheparinized blood or tiny blood clots are fed into it.

The result obtained will give a satisfactory capillary pH, base excess and bicarbonate. The carbon dioxide level is also representative although may be slightly higher than an arterial sample. The oxygen level however is not representative of the arterial oxygen concentration. The 'normal' capillary oxygen is about 5 kPa and if the result is much lower (<3 kPa) an arterial sample should be obtained.

BM stix test for blood glucose only requires one large drop of blood. The instructions on the container must be followed closely as the timing is critical for obtaining a reliable result.

Serum bilirubin estimation can be done with blood taken into a small capillary tube but it is wise to take some extra blood as these capillary tubes often disintegrate in the centrifuge.

Venous blood samples
Blood can be taken from any superficial vein. The usual sites are the back of the hand and the ankles or feet. The antecubital fossa can be used but can be difficult as the veins are set in loose tissue and may be mobile. Occasionally no vein is visible, but you still may be able to palpate a vein in which case you can take blood from it. Do not use the femoral vein. It is easy to go into the nearby hip joint in a baby and cause septic arthritis or osteomyelitis.

The easiest method is to use the 'broken-needle technique'. This may be slightly messy so put a paper towel on the cot to catch any loose drops of blood. The main advantage of this technique is that if the baby squirms and moves his arm, although you may lose a drop of blood, the needle stays in the vein and you can carry on with the sample collection. You will need:
• alcohol swab;
• 21G (green) needle;
• sample tubes;

- cotton-wool balls;
- tape.

Get everything ready with the blood bottles at hand. Snap the green hub off the needle shaft by repeatedly bending it (not much strength is required). Do not use smaller needles as the blood flows too slowly and the needle remains in the baby for a longer time.

Having found the vein, hold the baby's hand steadily in your left hand. Apply enough pressure to act as a tourniquet — do not squeeze too tightly as it is easy to overcome arterial pressure in a baby's limb and thus stop any blood flow to the vein. It is sometimes helpful to have your assistant hold the baby's limb higher up to steady it but make sure they are also not squeezing too tightly. The needle need only be inserted 2–3 mm into the vein and the blood should flow out quite quickly. Collect the drops into your tubes which must all be within reach.

Sometimes the blood comes out very slowly. Minor adjustments to the needle may remedy this, usually pulling it back a fraction or sometimes pushing it in further. Of course your adjustment may stop the blood flow altogether, so it may be better to be patient. Occasionally you have to give up with a particular vein as the flow stops altogether, but be ready as when you remove the needle, sometimes blood flows out of the hole in the skin. This happens when a small clot has blocked the lumen of the needle. The blood can be scooped into the bottle off the skin (although not for blood cultures).

When you have enough blood, remove the needle and simultaneously apply pressure to the puncture area with a cotton-wool ball which can be taped on when the bleeding has finished to keep the area clean. Make sure you do not leave the needle shaft on the cot and be sure to dispose of it correctly. Some people prefer to use a butterfly needle connected to a syringe rather than a broken needle. This has the advantage that there is less chance of blood being spilt. However it can be difficult as baby's veins are so fine that sucking back with the syringe easily collapses the vein and prevents blood flow.

Venous blood can also be collected at the time of inserting a cannula and this is described later.

Blood cultures require special techniques. If not carried out scrupulously there is a high rate of contamination, usually with skin commensals. The skin must be cleaned first with betadine. Ideally, the blood is taken using a butterfly needle. A minimum of 0.5 ml is necessary but you are more likely to isolate the organism if larger samples are obtained. Put a fresh needle on the syringe and put the blood into the blood culture bottles. The tinfoil caps should be removed at the last moment. Clean the rubber seal on the bottle with an alcohol wipe but allow it to dry before inserting the needle. Blood should be cultured in both an aerobic and anaerobic bottle. The bottles can be left in a warm incubator overnight.

As stated above, in practice it is not always possible to collect blood with a butterfly needle, especially in small babies. Using the broken-needle technique instead, the drops of blood can be collected straight into the top of a syringe that has had the plunger removed. You must first put a fine 25G (orange) needle on the other end of the syringe or the blood runs out. This orange needle can then be used for putting the blood into the culture bottles. You do not need the plunger as the blood will be sucked into the culture bottle which is under a vacuum.

A final method is to take blood with a green 21G needle without first snapping off the hub. As the blood appears, it can be sucked out of the hub into another sterile syringe and needle which can then be used to inject the blood into the culture bottles.

Arterial blood samples

If a blood gas estimation is required with an accurate oxygen and carbon dioxide concentration, an arterial blood sample is necessary. This can be obtained with an 'arterial stab' but once you have done this, it may be difficult to use that artery again for further samples as there will be bruising around the site. It is unlikely that only one sample will be necessary so if possible you should try to insert an arterial cannula. Even if you fail to insert the cannula, it is still likely that you will have obtained a sample and if you succeed, the line can be used for repeat sampling. The technique is described later but in the meanwhile, here is how to

do an arterial stab. You will need:
• alcohol swab;
• 25G (orange) needle;
• heparinized capillary tube;
• cotton-wool balls;
• tape.

The sample is usually taken from the radial artery. This can be felt at the wrist on the radial side of the forearm (the side with the thumb). It is often easier to use a fibreoptic cold light source. By shining this light through the baby's forearm from the other side, the artery can be identified. It is distinguishable from veins as it is so straight and runs parallel to the arm, it may also be seen to pulsate. You will not be able to transilluminate the artery in a fat baby.

Before putting a needle into the artery, you must test that the ulnar artery is present and also supplying blood to the hand. This is in case the radial artery is damaged or goes into spasm for any length of time, for without the ulnar artery the hand could become ischaemic. Simply press firmly to occlude the radial artery for 1–2 minutes. If the hand remains pink and warm then you know that the radial artery is not the only source of blood to the hand. Document that you have done this test in the notes.

Hold the baby's wrist in your left hand. The wrist should be held in an extended position at about 45°. If you over-extend it, the artery will be occluded. It is possible to hold the cold light in your left hand up against the back of the wrist at the same time, so that you can see the artery through the procedure.

Insert the orange needle directly into the artery at an angle less than 45° to the skin. Enter the skin just proximal to the transverse wrist crease. You can often feel a sudden give as it goes through the artery wall. Blood should flow back briskly and may be seen to pulsate. Collect the sample by holding the capillary tube up against the hub of the needle. Always collect a spare tube.

The commonest error is to insert the needle too far. Sometimes it goes into the artery then out the other side. The artery is more superficial than it seems and is usually only a few millimetres below the surface. So if blood does not flow back immediately, withdraw the needle a fraction at a time.

When you have enough blood, withdraw the needle and simultaneously apply firm pressure with a cotton-wool ball. This must be held in position for several minutes otherwise there will be a large bruise around the puncture site. When it stops bleeding, tape the cotton wool to the wrist.

If you are unsuccessful at collecting blood but have pierced the artery, then when you remove the needle blood will often flow onto the skin surface. This can still be collected in the capillary tube and used.

The other artery often used is the posterior tibial artery. It may be palpated between the medial malleolus of the ankle and the achilles tendon. You need to dorsiflex the foot otherwise the skin over the ankle is loose and wrinkled which makes aiming the needle impossible. The dorsalis pedis may also be tried. It is on the dorsum of the foot between the first and second metatarsal bones.

Do not use the femoral artery as you may damage the hip joint.

Inserting an IV cannula
With practice, you can put a cannula into almost any superficial vein in the body. Usual sites are the back of the hand, antecubital fossa, dorsum of the feet and medial side of the ankle (long saphenous vein). If you can not see a vein, it is worth checking behind the knee and the ventral side of the wrist. Even if you can not see the vein, it is often worth trying just in front of the medial malleolus for the long saphenous vein which is usually quite large. As a last resort, use one of the superficial veins on the scalp. You will have to shave some hair away otherwise you can not fix the cannula in place and most parents are unhappy about this. Do not use the veins on the forehead as if the vein blocks, extravasated infusion fluid can run into the loose space down as far as the eyebrows and this may lead to scalp necrosis with disastrous cosmetic consequences. You will need:
• alcohol swab;
• IV cannula 24G;
• T-connector;
• syringe with 2 ml 0.9% sodium chloride solution (saline);
• tape;

- cotton-wool balls;
- splint;
- bandage.

Get everything ready first. Cut the tape to the required lengths, connect the syringe to the T-connector and flush it through with the saline. Have everything to hand so that when you insert the cannula you can fix it in place quickly. If you are collecting blood at the same time, have all the sample bottles ready with the caps off. Finally check the needle moves freely out of the cannula as occasionally this is stiff at first.

It is easiest to insert a cannula with the baby lying on a flat surface such as a mattress. This way your left hand which is holding the baby's hand is also supported on the flat surface. It is inadvisable to attempt this procedure with the baby on the mother's or the nurse's lap.

Hold the relevant part of the baby in your left hand which acts as a tourniquet. Ask the assistant to help hold the baby and steady the limb without squeezing too hard.

Be confident and you will probably succeed. If conditions are not right, for example, the baby is not still enough, the vein you have selected has disappeared or there is not enough light, then wait and correct the situation. There is little point in just 'having a go' as you will fail. You lose confidence, the baby starts screaming and the parents become anxious.

Hold the skin taut over the vein, then insert the cannula directly into the vein, about 1–2 mm. You should immediately see blood flush back into the clear plastic part of the cannula. If not, do not give up yet, you may still be able to manouevre the cannula into the vein. When you have entered the vein, advance the cannula slowly and simultaneously remove the needle. Once the needle is out, you should see blood flow back into the plastic hub of the cannula. If you do not, it is unlikely that the cannula is still in the vein. However you can try flushing a small amount of the saline, if there is any resistance or a swelling appears under the skin then you have definitely missed the vein.

Tape the hub to the skin and if you are collecting blood, let it drip out of the hub into your sample bottles. Then connect the

T-connector to the hub and flush through 0.5–1 ml of the saline which should flow freely.

It is essential that you are certain that the cannula is properly in the vein. The superficial tissue of babies is very loose and modern syringe pumps will continue to push the fluid into the subcutaneous tissue if the cannula has come out of the vein. This can have serious consequences with certain infusions and drugs. Severe burns leading to necrosis and scarring, even permanent tendon damage may occur. Particularly notorious are solutions with high potassium content, calcium salts, high glucose concentrations and undiluted bicarbonate. Total parenteral nutrition given into a superficial vein can also be a problem if it extravasates.

With the T-connector in place, put a small piece of cotton-wool between the hub and the baby's skin as this is more comfortable for the baby. Tape the cannula securely, and fix the splint in place. Make sure the tape is not too tight otherwise it will occlude the vein and the infusion will stop working. Do not cover up the whole area so well that the nurses can not check the skin around the cannula to see whether the drip has tissued.

If you are unsuccessful, you should not have more than three attempts. After this it is unlikely that you will succeed with this particular baby and you must get help from a colleague. There is no shame and it is better to leave a few veins for someone else to have a try.

Umbilical vein cannulation
This is occasionally necessary in an emergency situation in the labour ward. It is described on p. 64.

Inserting an intra-arterial cannula
The method is very similar to doing an arterial stab, only instead of using a needle you use a standard intravenous cannula. Do not forget to check the radial artery is not the only arterial supply to the hand. You will need:
- alcohol swab;
- IV cannula 24G;

- T-connector;
- syringe with 2 ml heparinized 0.9% sodium chloride solution (1 unit heparin/1 ml of saline);
- tape;
- cotton-wool balls;
- splint;
- heparinized capillary tube.

There is no difference from an arterial stab in positioning the arm or inserting the cannula but it is much easier if you use a fibreoptic cold light as you insert the cannula. Once blood flushes back, slowly advance the cannula and remove the needle.

Quickly insert the T-connector into the hub or the baby can lose a lot of blood. Flush 0.5 ml heparinized saline slowly through the cannula. The skin over the area blanches transiently and this confirms you are in the artery and not a vein.

Secure the cannula and put a splint on the back of the wrist. Do not cover up the fingers and thumb. It is important to be able to see them to ensure that they have not become ischaemic. The digits must be checked every hour while the cannula is in place. If the tips of the fingers go white or blue the artery may be in spasm having just had the line inserted. This is usually transient but if there is no improvement after 10 minutes the cannula must be removed. If there is still some capillary return in the fingers and the colour seems to be improving, you can wait a little longer, however if the fingers are not completely normal by 30 minutes remove the line.

If you do not succeed in inserting the cannula, you still may be able to collect arterial blood off the skin surface so have a capillary tube nearby.

Once everything is in place, you should infuse 0.9% sodium chloride with heparin (1 unit/ml) at a rate of 0.2 ml/hour to ensure the line stays open.

Other possible sites to place an arterial line are the ulnar and the posterior tibial arteries. Never use the brachial artery as it is the sole supply to the lower arm. It is also better to avoid the femoral artery. Another artery that should not be cannulated is the superficial temporal artery on the side of the head. There is a risk of emboli or spasm affecting other branches of the external carotid artery.

LUMBAR PUNCTURE

Lumbar punctures are easier to perform in babies than in older children. The key to success is to get the baby in the correct position and to have an experienced nurse hold the baby in that position.

The baby will need to be on a firm surface and you need good light. You need:

* sterile paper towels;
* sterile rubber gloves;
* sterile paper sheet;
* betadine;
* clear antiseptic solution;
* cotton-wool balls;
* spinal needle (22G, 1.5 inches long);
* 4 sterile universal containers;
* 1 glucose bottle (yellow cap);
* collodion solution;
* sterile gauze;
* waterproof tape.

Before washing your hands, get the baby in the right position and take off the nappy. Lie him on his left side so that his head is to your left when you sit down. He must be curled into a flexed fetal position. This must not be overdone as it may impede his breathing, and you must be gentle with a sick baby. It is important that his spine remains parallel to the surface he is lying on (Fig. 22.3a). The baby will tend to flex his spine laterally by lifting his bottom off the bed, particularly when the needle is inserted. It is helpful if a second assistant keeps a hand on his bottom to stop it lifting as the prime holder will not be able to prevent this. The other important thing about the position is to have the plane of his back at 90° to the bed to avoid rotation of the spine (Fig. 22.3b).

In the newborn the spinal cord ends at the level of the third

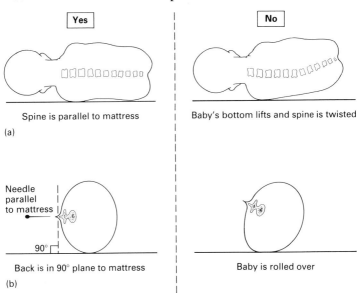

Fig. 22.3 Position of the baby for a lumbar puncture. (a) Baby's back. (b) 'Cross-section' of baby.

lumbar vertebra (in adults it ends higher at the lower border of the first lumbar vertebra). The landmark is the right iliac crest, feel for the tubercle of the crest which is the highest point palpable. If you drop a vertical line down from this point, it crosses the spine through the fourth lumbar vertebra or through the space between the fourth and fifth lumbar vertebrae. This is where to insert the needle (Fig. 22.4). It is worth marking this with a pen before you start.

Wash your hands with liquid soap or antiseptic. Put on the rubber gloves, a mask is optional. Put the sterile sheet under the baby and check his position is correct.

Clean the area on his back carefully with the betadine, wiping down towards his bottom but not up again. It is worth putting some betadine over the iliac crest so that you can feel this later if you want to check your landmark. Use the clear antiseptic to wipe off the betadine over the spine so that you get a clear view. Cover his bottom with a sterile towel.

Check the baby's position again and that everyone is ready.

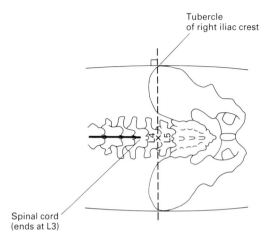

Fig. 22.4 Anatomical landmarks for a lumbar puncture. Drop a vertical line from tubercle of right iliac crest. The line crosses the spinal column through body of L4 or the L4/5 space. The needle should be inserted in the first space caudal to this line. X marks the position to insert needle.

The needle is held so that you can see the bevelled edge and the tip of the trocar is facing you, this will mean the ligaments are split rather than torn.

Having felt the space between the vertebrae again, insert the needle through the overlying skin. The needle must go in parallel to the bed, at 90° to the plane of the baby's back. Aim between the spines towards the umbilicus. The needle passes through skin, subcutaneous tissue, spinal ligaments, epidural space and finally through the dura into the subarachnoid space where the cerebrospinal fluid (CSF) is situated. It need only go in 1 cm in the newborn to reach the subarachnoid space (5–7 mm in a preterm baby) and you may feel a 'pop' or 'give' as it passes through the dura. This is not always obvious and it is easy to go too far. Unfortunately you then hit the vertebral venous plexus and blood flows back making the specimen of CSF heavily bloodstained.

If you feel a grinding sensation you have hit the spine itself. If it is just under the skin, it will be the spinous process and this usually means the spine is twisted or rotated so remove the needle and reposition the baby. It could be that you have gone right through the subarachnoid space and hit the vertebral body, in which case withdraw the needle slightly.

When you think you are in the subarachnoid space, remove the trocar from the hollow cannula. CSF should flow back but may take a few seconds to appear. If CSF does not drip out, adjust the needle, inserting it a few mm further or try withdrawing it slightly.

When you are successful, collect a few drops in three containers which should be numbered in order, and a few drops in the glucose bottle. No more than 1 ml total CSF needs be taken. The fourth container is spare but useful to have handy as an empty container often falls off the trolley. Send the second bottle to the biochemistry laboratory (protein and glucose) and the other two bottles to the microbiology laboratory.

When you have enough CSF and all the caps have been screwed tightly on the bottles, remove the needle. This is done in one clean action then press on the area firmly with some sterile gauze. Put some collodion solution on some gauze and put this over the puncture site. This gauze should be fixed in place with waterproof tape so that if the baby has a dirty nappy later the area can not become contaminated.

Finally, make sure that all the betadine is cleaned off the baby as iodine can be absorbed through the baby's thin skin. Do not forget to take a blood sample for glucose at the same time otherwise the CSF glucose result can not be interpreted. Record the whole procedure in the baby's notes.

A hollow needle (without a trocar) should not be used to penetrate the skin as there is a risk of pushing a tiny piece of skin into the dural area which may result in an implantation dermoid cyst forming. In time this can grow and compress the spinal cord.

COLLECTING URINE

However you collect urine, if microscopy and culture are required, it must be sent to the microbiologist immediately. Leaving a sample overnight, even in a refrigerator, can lead to bacterial contamination of the specimen and give misleading results.

Bag urines

These should not be used if the urine is not required for microbiological purposes, but can be used for tests such as electrolytes, osmolality or amino acid chromatography. Make sure the bag is sealed properly or urine will leak out of the bag. The skin must be dry and free from cream otherwise the bag will not stay in place.

Clean-catch urine

This can be very time-consuming but is necessary in order to obtain a urine sample that is not contaminated. The baby's genital area should be cleaned first with sterile water (which itself sometimes stimulates the baby to pass urine). Someone then has to sit and wait until the baby passes urine and catch the free flow into a sterile container. 1 ml of urine is sufficient for microscopy and culture. It is relatively easy with a boy but baby girls can be difficult as the urine tends to dribble rather than spurt out.

Another technique to encourage the baby to pass urine is to hold him in the ventral suspension position (see Fig. 7.4) and gently stroke his back parallel to the lumbar spine.

Suprapubic aspirate (SPA)

It is sometimes necessary to collect urine directly from the bladder and this is the most reliable way of obtaining a non-contaminated specimen. Inserting a urinary catheter to collect a specimen is not recommended in babies so urine must be aspirated with a needle.

Never attempt this if the baby has a wet nappy as the bladder will probably be empty. Ideally an SPA is done under ultrasound control as you can be sure that there is urine in the bladder and you have a guide where to aim the needle. You need:
- betadine;
- cotton-wool balls;
- sterile gloves;
- 10 ml syringe;
- 23G (blue) needle;
- sterile container;
- elastoplast.

Wash your hands and put on the gloves then clean around the baby's lower abdominal wall with antiseptic and dry the area. The cold antiseptic may stimulate the baby to pass urine spontaneously so have the container at hand.

The baby should lie on his back on a firm surface and the assistant must hold the child firmly so he can not struggle.

The bladder is an abdominal organ in the newborn and you do not enter the peritoneal cavity so it is a safe procedure. However it should not be done in infants over the age of 6 months.

Insert the needle 1 cm above the symphysis pubis in the midline. Aim it directly downwards towards the mattress and not at an angle into the pelvis. This ensures you enter the bladder through the dome which contains no pain fibres. If you aim towards the pelvis you may hit the trigone of the bladder which is extremely painful.

As you push the needle down into the bladder pull back slightly on the plunger of the syringe. This creates negative pressure so that as soon as you are in the bladder, urine will be aspirated into the syringe. If you do not do this, there is a risk that you will not realize you are in the bladder and go through the far side. Then you may penetrate intestine lying posterior to the bladder. It is usually sufficient to insert the needle 1–2 cm and you should not insert it more than 2 cm.

Once you have obtained 1 ml of urine, remove the needle. Press over the puncture site with cotton-wool then put an elastoplast over the area.

If there is time, it is kinder to put some lignocaine cream (EMLA) on the baby's skin first. This takes 1 hour to take effect.

PASSING A NASOGASTRIC TUBE

The technique is described on p. 144. If you want a sample of gastric aspirate, simply place 2 ml of stomach contents into a sterile container.

INTUBATING A BABY

See Chapter 5, p. 59.

Appendix

1: Centile Charts for Birthweight and Head Circumference

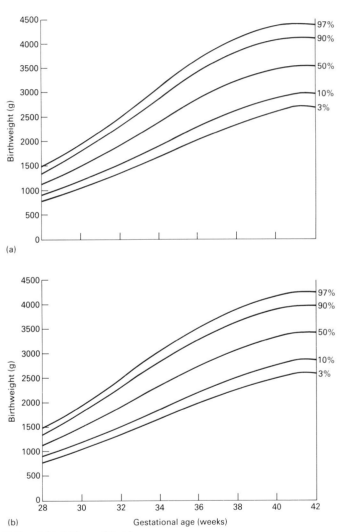

Birthweight (a) boys; (b) girls.

Charts adapted from Yudkin PL, Aboualfa M, Eyre JA, Redman CWG & Wilkinson AR (1987) New birthweight and head circumference centiles for gestational ages 24 to 42 weeks. *Early Human Development*, **15**: 45–52. © Castlemead Publications, chart refs 87 and 88.

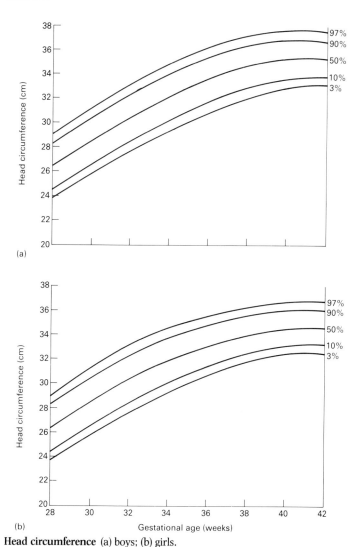

Head circumference (a) boys; (b) girls.

2: Mortality Rates

Stillbirth rate is the number of stillborn babies (over 28 weeks gestation per 1000 total births.

Neonatal mortality rate is the number of babies who die within the first 28 days of life per 1000 live births. This is divided into *early* (0–7 days) and *late* (8–28 days).

Perinatal mortality rate is the stillbirth rate added to the early neonatal mortality rate per 1000 total births.

Infant mortality rate is the number of babies who die in the first year of life per 1000 live births.

Postneonatal mortality rate is the number of babies who die after the neonatal period (>28 days) but within the first year per 1000 live births. Sudden infant death syndrome contributes almost half the mortality of this group.

The following are figures obtained from the Office of Population Censuses and Surveys (OPCS) for England & Wales.

Mortality rates	1985	1990
Stillbirth rate	5.5	4.6
Neonatal mortality rate	5.3	4.6
Early	4.3	3.5
Late	1.0	1.1
Perinatal mortality rate	9.8	8.1
Infant mortality rate	9.2	7.9
Postneonatal mortality rate	3.9	3.3

The figures continue to show a gradual fall apart from the late neonatal mortality rate.

Mortality rates vary with maternal age (increased in mothers under 20 and over 35 years), as well as parity, social class, place of birth and region of residence of the mother.

3: Neonatal Reflexes

Testing for neonatal reflexes does not usually form part of the routine examination of the newborn. However they should be assessed if there is evidence of a neurological abnormality or there has been a potential insult to the brain. The reflexes may also be a guide to gestational age of a premature baby and a table is given of the gestational age at which some of the reflexes may be seen.

Reflexes	Expected onset (completed weeks gestation)
Pupil reaction to light	29–31
Glabellar tap	32–34
Traction	33–36
Neck righting	34–37
Head turning to diffuse light	32–36

Taking the example of the reaction of the pupils to light, if this is present then the baby is more than 29 weeks, whereas if this is absent then the baby is less than 31 weeks gestation.

Glabellar tap. A gentle tap on the glabella (the junction between the nose and forehead) causes blinking of the eyelids on both sides.

Traction (Trunk elevation). While lying on his back, the baby is pulled upwards holding his wrists. The trunk is thus raised from the supine position, and the neck flexors contract and prevent the head from falling backwards.

Neck righting. If the head is turned passively onto one side, the whole trunk follows.

Moro response. The infant is placed on his back with his head resting on one of the examiner's palms about 1–3 cm above the mattress. The head must be in the midline. The hand is rapidly dropped down 1–2 cm allowing the head to fall backwards. This test should be performed gently. Explain first to the parents what you are about to do as it looks rather alarming. As the head falls back, the arms are abducted and extended. This is followed by adduction of the arms like a hug. The test may need to be repeated two to three times to elicit the response. The reflex is sometimes seen if the baby is startled by a sharp tap on the cot but the head must be in the midline for the test to be valid.

Palmar grasp. A finger placed in the palm from the ulnar side causes the baby to flex his fingers and grip the examiner's finger. Take care not to touch the back of the baby's hand as this may inhibit the grasp response. If the examiner raises his finger slowly there is progressive increase in tone of the baby's arm muscles allowing the baby to be lifted momentarily.

Rooting. When the infant's cheek touches the mother's breast this reflex enables him to find the nipple. When the corner of the infant's mouth is touched, the head and tongue turn towards the stimulus and the lip lowers on the same side.

Crossed extension. The sole of one foot is stroked while holding the leg extended at the knee. The opposite leg flexes, adducts and then extends as if to push away an irritating object.

Automatic walking. The infant is held upright supported under his arms. Pressure on the sole of one foot on the table is followed by flexion of the opposite leg. The alternating flexion and extension of the legs resembles walking.

4: Dubowitz Scheme
for Gestational Assessement

This method for assessing gestational age should only be carried out when the baby is between 6 and 24 hours of age. It relies on the superficial appearance of the baby as well as neurological criteria. The age given is a guide only.

Neuro-logical sign	Score					
	0	1	2	3	4	5
Posture						
Square window	90°	60°	45°	30°	0°	
Ankle dorsi-flexion	90°	75°	45°	20°	0°	
Arm recoil	180°	90–180°	<90°			
Leg recoil	180°	90–180°	<90°			
Popliteal angle	180°	160°	130°	110°	90°	<90°
Heel to ear						
Scarf sign						
Head lag						
Ventral suspen-sion						

Neurological criteria (See also notes on p. 275).

271

External (superficial) criteria

External sign	Score				
	0	1	2	3	4
Oedema	Obvious oedema hands and feet, pitting over tibia	No obvious oedema hands and feet; pitting over tibia	No oedema		
Skin texture	Very thin, gelatinous	Thin and smooth	Smooth; medium thickness. Rash or superficial peeling	Slight thickening. Superficial cracking and peeling esp. hands and feet	Thick and parchment-like, superficial or deep cracking
Skin colour (infant not crying)	Dark red	Uniformly pink	Pale pink: variable over body	Pale. Only pink over ears, lips, palms or soles	
Skin opacity (trunk)	Numerous veins and venules clearly seen, especially over abdomen	Veins and tributaries seen	A few large vessels clearly seen over abdomen	A few large vessels seen indistinctly over abdomen	No blood vessels seen
Lanugo (over back)	No lanugo	Abundant: long and thick over whole back	Hair thinning especially over lower back	Small amount of lanugo and bald areas	At least half of back devoid of lanugo
Breast size	No breast tissue palpable	Breast tissue on one or both sides <0.5 cm diameter	Breast tissue both sides; one or both 0.5–1.0 cm	Breast tissue both sides; one or both >1 cm	

Plantar creases	No skin creases	Faint red marks over anterior half of sole	Definite red marks over more than anterior half: indentations over less than anterior third	Indentations over more than anterior third	Definite deep indentations over more than anterior third
Nipple formation	Nipple barely visible; no areola	Nipple well defined; areola smooth and flat; diameter <0.75 cm	Areola stippled, edge not raised; diameter <0.75 cm	Areola stippled, edge raised; diameter >0.75 cm	
Ear form	Pinna flat and shapeless, little or no incurving of edge	Incurving of part of edge of pinna	Partial incurving whole of upper pinna	Well-defined incurving whole of upper pinna	
Ear firmness	Pinna soft, easily folded, no recoil	Pinna soft, easily folded, slow recoil	Cartilage to edge of pinna, but soft in places, ready recoil	Pinna firm, cartilage to edge, instant recoil	
Genitalia males females (with hips half abducted)	Neither testis in scrotum Labia majora widely spearated, labia minora protruding	At least one testis high in scrotum Labia majora almost cover labia minora	At least one testis right down Labia majora completely cover labia minora		

Graph for reading gestational age from total score
The total score for the neurological criteria (see p. 271) and the external criteria (see p. 272) are added together and the gestational age is read on the graph below.

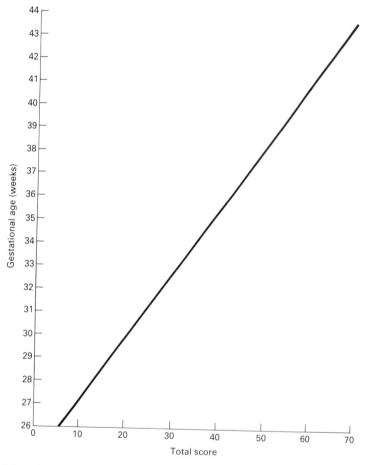

Adapted with permission from Dubowitz LMS, Dubowitz V & Goldberg C (1970). Clinical assessment of gestational age in the newborn infant. *Journal of Pediatrics*, **77**: 1–10.

Some notes on techniques of assessment of neurological criteria

Posture. Observed with infant quiet and in supine position. Score 0: arms and legs extended; 1: beginning of flexion of hips and knees, arms extended; 2: stronger flexion of legs, arms extended; 3: arms slightly flexed, legs flexed and abducted; 4: full flexion of arms and legs.

Square window. The hand is flexed on the forearm between the thumb and index finger of the examiner. Enough pressure is applied to get as full a flexion as possible, and the angle between the hypothenar eminence and the ventral aspect of the forearm is measured and graded according to diagram. (Care is taken not to rotate the infant's wrist while doing this manoeuvre.)

Ankle dorsiflexion. The foot is dorsiflexed onto the anterior aspect of the leg, with the examiner's thumb on the sole of the foot and other fingers behind the leg. Enough pressure is applied to get as full flexion as possible, and the angle between the dorsum of the foot and the anterior aspect of the leg is measured.

Arm recoil. With the infant in the supine position the forearms are first flexed for 5 seconds, then fully extended by pulling on the hands, and then released. The sign is fully positive if the arms return briskly to full flexion (Score 2). If the arms return to incomplete flexion or the response is sluggish it is graded as Score 1. If they remain extended or are only followed by random movements the score is 0.

Leg recoil. With the infant supine, the hips and knees are fully flexed for 5 seconds, then extended by traction on the feet, and released. A maximal response is one of full flexion of the hips and knees (Score 2). A partial flexion scores 1, and minimal or no movement scores 0.

Popliteal angle. With the infant supine and his pelvis flat on the examining couch, the thigh is held in the knee-chest position by the examiner's left index finger and thumb supporting the knee. The leg is then extended by gentle pressure from the examiner's right index finger behind the ankle and the popliteal angle is measured.

Heel-to-ear manoeuvre. With the baby supine, draw the baby's foot as near to the head as it will go without forcing it. Observe the distance between the foot and the head as well as the degree of extension at the knee. Grade according to diagram. Note that the knee is left free and may draw down alongside the abdomen.

Scarf sign. With the baby supine, take the infant's hand and try to put it around the neck and as far posteriorly as possible around the opposite shoulder. Assist this manoeuvre by lifting the elbow across the body. See how far the elbow will go across and grade accordingly to illustrations. Score 0 : elbow reaches opposite axillary line; 1: elbow between midline and opposite axillary line; 2: elbow reaches midline; 3: elbow will not reach midline.

Head lag. With the baby lying supine, grasp the hands (or the arms if a very small infant) and pull him slowly towards the sitting position. Observe the position of the head in relation to the trunk and grade accordingly. In a small infant the head may initially be supported by one hand. Score 0: complete lag; 1 partial head control; 2: able to maintain head in line with body; 3: brings head anterior to body.

Ventral suspension. The infant is suspended in the prone position, with examiner's hand under the infant's chest (one hand in a small infant, two in a large infant). Observe the degree of extension of the back and the amount of flexion of the arms and legs. Also note the relation of the head to the trunk. Grade according to diagrams.

   If score differs on the two sides, take the mean.

5: Phototherapy Charts

These charts give a guide as to the necessity of treating a jaundiced baby with phototherapy. Different charts exist for different gestational ages and the acceptable level of serum bilirubin depends upon the baby's age from birth.

Phototherapy is required if the serum bilirubin lies above the line.

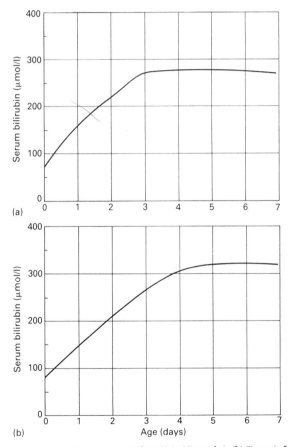

Phototherapy charts (a) Preterm infant (34–37 weeks). (b) Term infant (37 + weeks).

6: Guthrie Test

Every baby in the UK undergoes screening on the sixth day of life for phyenylketonuria (PKU) and congenital hypothyroidism. Four drops of blood are taken by the midwife using a heel-prick and placed on the circles in the card which is shown opposite. The baby must be on normal milk feeds (breast or formula milk) and if intake is inadequate, the test must be delayed until full feeds are being given.

Phenylketonuria is a rare autosomal recessive metabolic disease in which lack of a particular enzyme leads to a build up of phenylalanine in the body. Once diagnosed, the infants must be given a special diet otherwise permanent brain damage is sustained, hence the importance of screening.

Screening for congenital hypothyroidism is also carried out on this card as it may be difficult to diagnose clinically in the neonatal period (see p. 116). Blood spots are analysed for TSH (thyroid-stimulating hormone) and thyroxine.

Biochemical screening for cystic fibrosis is also possible using the blood spots on the Guthrie card but this is not current practice in the UK.

NEONATAL SCREENING BLOOD TEST
Complete all sections of this form legibly using ball point pen

Surname			
First name			
Address			
Mothers first name			

Birth Wt.	kg	Sex	M ☐ F ☐

Please tick if repeat test ☐		District	

Date	D	M	Y	Community/Hospital
Birth				

Specimen	GP/Consultant

First Milk Feed	Address of GP or Hospital

Name of Health Visitor or Midwife	

Phenylketonuria

☐ Normal result

☐ Further test required
see comment

Hypothyroidism

☐ Normal result

☐ Further test required
see comment

COMMENT

Fill each circle completely with ONE DROP of blood to soak through to back of card. Allow to dry.

HMR 101/6

Printed in the UK for HMSO 4/90 Dd 8260343 C5,280 (11037)

Guthrie card. Reproduced by permission of the Registrar General for England and Wales and the Controller of Her Majesty's Stationery Office.

7: Initial Immunization Schedule

The schedule for routine immunization has changed recently and is now started earlier, at 2 months of age. In addition, immunization against *Haemophilus influenzae* is available from October 1992. The following are now given in the first 2 years of life:

Immunization	Schedule
Diphtheria Tetanus Pertussis *Haemophilus influenzae* Oral polio	Primary course given at 2, 3 and 4 months
Measles/mumps/rubella	Given at 12–18 months
BCG	May be given to infants under certain circumstances (see p. 17)

Preterm babies are immunized at the appropriate chronological age (i.e. age from birth), regardless of their gestational age at birth. Live oral polio vaccine should not be given until the baby leaves the neonatal unit.

It is the responsibility of the person administering the vaccine to check whether there are any contraindications. However certain situations in the neonatal period may lead to the need for special assessment as to the suitability of pertussis vaccination. These include:

1 Documented history of cerebral damage in the neonatal period.
2 Neonatal convulsions.

The presence of these relative contraindications must be passed on to the general practitioner in the baby's discharge summary from hospital.

It should be stressed that the following neonatal situations are *not* contraindications to pertussis vaccination:
• breastfeeding;
• neonatal jaundice;
• low birthweight (including prematurity);

• stable neurological conditions such as cerebral palsy and Down's syndrome.

Further information can be obtained in the following guide: Department of Health (1992) *Immunization Against Disease*. Department of Health,Whitehall, London.

8: Sleeping Position of Infants

In November 1991, the Department of Health issued recommendations on the sleeping position of infants to try to reduce the incidence of cot death (Sudden Infant Death Syndrome). This followed assessment of several studies conducted around the world (including the UK).

Babies should no longer be placed prone (on their front) when they are laid down to sleep. They should be placed either on their back (supine) or on their sides.

Despite previous teaching, there is no evidence that placing healthy babies on their back results in an increased risk of death from choking or vomiting.

There are, however, certain circumstances in which the babies should be nursed prone. These include some babies in neonatal units, babies with severe gastro-oesophageal reflux, babies receiving treatment in splints for unstable hips, and babies with Pierre Robin syndrome.

By 6–7 months of age, many babies will roll themselves over onto their front during sleep. There is no need for concern over this as the incidence of cot death is markedly reduced by this age.

9: Audiological Screening

All babies will be screened for hearing problems during developmental checks carried out at 8 months. However certain babies should be referred for audiological screening before 3 months of age. The following are some indications:

1 Low birthweight (<1.5 kg).
2 Family history of deafness in childhood.
3 Congenital infections (e.g. rubella, CMV, toxoplasma).
4 Head or neck malformations (particularly cleft palate).
5 Severe hyperbilirubinaemia requiring exchange transfusion.
6 Meningitis and severe neonatal sepsis.
7 Birth asphyxia.
8 Toxic blood gentamicin levels.
9 Congenital hypothyroidism.
10 Parental consanguinity.

In addition if parents are convinced their baby can not hear then the baby's hearing should be checked.

10: Circumcision

Most circumcisions are performed for religious reasons. Jewish boys are circumcised on the eighth day of life and Moslem boys between the ages of 3 and 15 years.

If the baby is born with hypospadias (see p. 97), the circumcision should not performed as the foreskin is needed for the corrective operation.

Parents sometimes ask a paediatrician whether the baby should be circumcised for medical reasons. Routine circumcision is practiced in the USA but is not common in the UK. We have outlined below the arguments both for and against routine circumcision.

BENEFITS

1 *Cancer of the penis* is almost abolished in circumcised males. However this is a rare condition even among uncircumcised men.

2 *Sexually transmitted diseases* are more common in uncircumcised men.

3 *Cancer of the cervix* was thought to be more common in wives of uncircumcised men. However, this may be related to the passage of viruses that are associated with cervical cancer.

4 *Genital hygiene* is improved after circumcision as many organisms colonize the skin under the prepuce. However regular washing with soap and water in the bath is also effective unless adhesions prevent retraction of the foreskin. It should be stressed here that no attempt should be made to retract the foreskin until the child is at least 4 years old. Earlier attempts may damage the mucosa which heals by fibrosis and scarring. This leads to permanent adhesions that will necessitate circumcision during adolescence.

5 *Phimosis* (gross narrowing of the preputial orifice) can obviously not occur in circumcised boys but is uncommon unless the foreskin is forcibly retracted as described above.

6 *Urinary tract infection* is more common in uncircumcised

infants, due to the increased presence of periurethral bacteria that can cause ascending infection of the urinary tract.

RISKS

1 *Pain* is certainly felt by babies and circumcision without anaesthesia is extremely painful. It is impossible to say whether there are any long-term psychological effects on the baby although this is unlikely.

2 *Bleeding* may occur after circumcision, particularly if the baby did not receive vitamin K at birth.

3 *Infection* of the wound is unusual but also a potential complication of circumcision.

4 *Scarring* is unusual and only occurs if the circumcision is performed badly.

CONCLUSION

The only medical indication for routine circumcision would seem to be prevention of urinary tract infection. Although the risks of circumcision are small, the benefits are not convincing and we would not recommend this as routine practice.

Occasionally therapeutic circumcision is necessary if the infant has recurrent purulent balanitis (inflammation of the glans penis) or ballooning of the foreskin at the beginning of micturition due to phimosis.

11: Comparison Table of Gauges

Throughout the text we have used French catheter gauge size when describing sizes of tubes. This is common usage in the UK but below are equivalent sizes in millimetres.

French catheter gauge	Diameter in mm
3	1.0
4	1.33
5	1.67
6	2.0
7	2.33
8	2.67
9	3.0
10	3.33
11	3.67
12	4.0
13	4.33
14	4.67
15	5.0
16	5.33

12: Recommended Reading

Gandy GM & Roberton NRC (1987) *Lecture Notes on Neonatology.* Blackwell Scientific Publications, Oxford.

Roberton NRC (1988) *A Manual of Normal Neonatal Care.* Edward Arnold, London.

Thomas R & Harvey D (1992) *Colour Guide: Neonatology.* Churchill Livingstone, Edinburgh.

Valman HB (1989) *The First Year of Life.* British Medical Association, London.

Index